A SHORT HISTORY OF MEDICINE

ERWIN H. ACKERKNECHT (M.D., Leipzig, 1931; M.D.h.c., Bern, 1976, Geneva, 1978; Diploma in Ethnology, Paris, 1939) served in the French and British armies in 1940. He came to the United States in 1941 as a Fellow at The Johns Hopkins University (Member of the Society of Scholars, 1981). From 1947 to 1957 he was professor of the history of medicine at the University of Wisconsin, Madison. From 1957 until his retirement in 1971 he was professor of the history of medicine at the University of Zurich, where he is emeritus director of the Institute of Medical History. Dr. Ackerknecht's many writings on the history of medicine include *Medicine at the Paris Hospital, 1794–1848* (Johns Hopkins Press, 1967), a biography of Rudolph Virchow, and a history of therapeutics.

A SHORT HISTORY OF MEDICINE

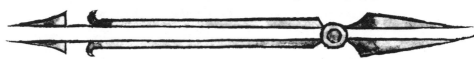

Erwin H. Ackerknecht, M.D.

Revised Edition

THE JOHNS HOPKINS UNIVERSITY PRESS

Baltimore and London

Originally published in English as *A Short History of Medicine*, by
the Ronald Press Company, New York, 1955. Revised edition, 1968.

Originally published in German as *Geschichte der Medizin*, by
Ferdinand Enke Verlag, 1959. Copyright © 1959, 1979 by Ferdinand Enke Verlag, Stuttgart

Johns Hopkins Paperbacks edition, revised, 1982
01 00 99 98 97 96 95 94   10 9 8 7

The Johns Hopkins University Press
2715 North Charles Street
Baltimore, Maryland 21218-4319
The Johns Hopkins Press Ltd., London

Library of Congress Cataloging in Publication Data

Ackerknecht, Erwin Heinz, 1906–
 A short history of medicine.

 Reprint. Originally published: Rev. print.
New York: Ronald Press Co., 1968.
 Bibliography: p. 245
 Includes index.
 1. Medicine—History. I. Title.   [DNLM:
1. History of medicine. WZ 40 A182s]
R131.A34   1982   610′.9   81–48194
ISBN 0–8018–2726–4 (pbk.)   AACR2

Cover illustration: Surgical instruments, from Hans von Gersdorff's *Feldtbuch der Wundartzney*, Strassburg, 1540
Design: Susan P. Fillion

A Catalog record for this book is available from the British
Library.

To
PAUL CRANEFIELD
and
CHARLES ROSENBERG

CONTENTS

CONTENTS

ILLUSTRATIONS

PREFACE TO FIRST EDITION

Long experience in teaching and with medical practitioners has convinced me of the need for a short, yet systematic, history of medicine suitable for those who wish to familiarize themselves with the field without wading through extensive and detailed treatises. Written to meet this need, the present work is designed to be of service to the medical student, the busy doctor, and other members of the great health team, as well as to educated laymen interested in health problems.

I have compressed into twenty short chapters the fascinating story of man's progress in the science and art of medicine. This story begins with the first groping attempts of primitive man to fight disease with magic and stone knives. It goes on to describe the medical activities of the early civilizations of Egypt, Asia, and America; the accomplishments of the great authorities of classical antiquity from Hippocrates to Galen; the stagnation of the Middle Ages; and the progress that followed the renaissance of medicine in the sixteenth century. Particular attention is then paid to the rapid developments of the nineteenth century. A special chapter is devoted to the history of medicine in the United States, and the book concludes with a short survey of present-day achievements throughout the world. Though in the abstract the period since 1800 is no more important than many other ages, to the modern reader it is incomparably more meaningful and accessible.

My aim has been to orient the reader to the bewildering problems of medicine in the present and future by recapturing the triumphs and difficulties of the past. By its very nature, a treatment of this sort must be selective. I have concentrated on clarifying the main lines of development, deliberately avoiding the mere cataloguing of individual accomplishments. Important names have been treated primarily as symbols for groups of men all working in the same direction. Some of the names omitted are as significant in themselves as many of those mentioned; but they do not serve so well to represent the main currents of medical progress. With the same objective in view I have tried to strike a reasonable balance between the history of medicine proper and its social and cultural background, between medical science and medical practice, and between clinical and preventive medicine.

The selection of suggested readings at the end of the book has been guided by considerations of a purely functional nature. The references selected are those which will help the reader toward a better understanding of the text; they are in no sense a compendious listing of the sources I myself have used. All are readily obtainable in most libraries, and all are available in English. Since it is my considered opinion that nobody really understands medical history unless he has read at least a few of the original texts, I have made a serious effort to list reprints and translations of medical classics.

A book of this type must necessarily draw on many sources, not all of which can be acknowledged in detail in the limited space available. Of the general histories of medicine, I have profited most from those of Fielding H. Garrison, Max Neuburger, and Charles Daremberg. I have also learned much from Johann Hermann Baas, Julius Pagel, Carl Wunderlich, and Heinrich Haeser. I have been particularly instructed and stimulated throughout the years by my teacher, the late Henry E. Sigerist, and two friends and colleagues, Owsei Temkin and the late George Rosen. As for other sources of information and inspiration, I have to omit with regret the names of many respected colleagues in medicine, history, and anthropology, and, last but not least, my students, especially those who have worked with me in seminars and on doctoral theses. I alone am responsible for errors and misconceptions.

The history of medicine does not lack dark pages. Yet as a whole it is considerably more encouraging than the history of many other human activities. It is full of interesting events and valuable lessons. I dare to hope that with all its limitations this book will evoke in the reader at least some of the fascination and enthusiasm which its author has experienced in studying the long road which man has trodden in his fight against disease.

ERWIN H. ACKERKNECHT

Madison, Wisconsin
June, 1955

PREFACE, 1982 EDITION

The need for a text of this type continues, as has been shown by the appearance of new and revised editions of this book in several languages. It gives me particular pleasure that The Johns Hopkins University Press, which in 1945 published my first book in the United States (*Malaria in the Upper Mississippi Valley, 1760–1900*), has decided to bring out a revised edition of the English-language version.

I have not changed the basic plan or structure of the book, as they seem to serve their purpose in a satisfactory way. I have made numerous additions and corrections, however, particularly in the second half of the book. These are necessitated by advances in our medical and historical knowledge and insight and, above all, by the extremely rapid evolution of medicine during the last two decades.

In republishing this little text, I feel a deep sense of gratitude to the United States, the country that forty years ago adopted me, a lonely refugee, and thus became my country and that of my children and grandchildren.

E.H.A

Zurich
July, 1981

WHY MEDICAL HISTORY?

There are many ways to study medical history and many reasons for such a study. Some study it in order to gain a better understanding of history in general. Medicine and disease have had an undeniable effect on the whole of history, and the medical behavior of a period can be regarded as a kind of projective test of the total culture of that period. We know much more about a society when we know how it treated its sick and what it thought disease to be.

But perhaps the most usual reason for studying medical history is the desire to understand medicine itself and to grasp its techniques, its organization, and its underlying ideas. The desire and need to understand medicine is not confined to the medical profession. It is of personal concern to the object of medical practice—the patient. And virtually everyone is a patient today. We live in a period in which, as Galdston says, "we have converted mortality into morbidity." Yet, while the average person now gets far more medical attention than in any previous period, it is paradoxical that the meaning of disease and its treatment is even more obscure to him than to his ancestors.

The medical systems of earlier times are instructive both in their similarities and in their dissimilarities to the medicine of today. Though these systems differed profoundly from our own, it must always be remembered that they functioned, that they fulfilled their task. Studying the history of medicine from this point of view has an illuminating and sobering effect and takes away a little from the smugness of the proud citizen of the hydrogen-bomb age. On the other hand, in spite of all the unfamiliar theories and techniques, the medicine of former periods has many important similarities to our own system. Most of the problems were the same. The study of how solutions were approached, obtained, or missed in the past helps in finding, or at least understanding, the solutions of our own time. Parallel to discontinuity there runs a great continuity in the history of medicine. Answers given to problems today become more intelligible when they are seen as the continuation of answers given in former times.

One of the great obstacles to an understanding of modern medicine is its complexity, its incredible wealth of seemingly unrelated details. This complexity has led to specialization, which in turn has further intensified the complexity. There is no better way than the study of medical history to bring some order and coherence into this oppressive mass of details. As the details are ordered historically, the fundamental ideas that govern modern medical thinking and action begin to stand out; and the observer is enabled to apply them to the modern picture. The student of medicine must grasp the role of anatomy in the growth of medicine since Vesalius, the periodic victories of the chemical approach, the part played by the laboratory in clinical medicine since the middle of the last century, and the recurrent idea that the healing force of nature can be replaced by the curative activities of the physician. Only then will he have a clear understanding of the essential features and trends of present-day medicine. As the only discipline that presents medicine as a whole, medical history is a valuable antidote to certain mental attitudes growing out of the unavoidable specialization of which medical men rightly complain.

Medical men are accustomed to analyzing the organism historically by means of embryology and to determining the status of their patients through case histories. But when it comes to understanding their own craft they, and the laymen who necessarily follow them, are liable to forego the historical approach. They live, thus, with the misconception that every good thought and useful technique was invented only yesterday and that most important problems are very close to final solution. The widespread absence of real understanding is reflected in the continuous use of such expressions as "miracle drug" or "miraculous operation," which underlines the fact that at heart many of our contemporaries feel themselves to be surrounded by a magic universe, just as their Stone Age or medieval ancestors did. In historical perspective medicine loses its miraculous quality. It remains complex and fascinating, but it becomes an understandable phenomenon.

Medical history is often accused of dealing with "old theories." This reproach overlooks the fact that modern medicine, too, depends upon certain basic philosophical assumptions and scientific theories, even though it may not formulate them as clearly as its predecessors. These will be the "old theories" of tomorrow. Modern men, no less than men of former times, see only what they are prepared to see, and a new outlook is always needed in order to see something fundamentally new. Therefore it is a most valuable feature of medical history that it makes us conscious of the important role of theories, for better or worse, at all times. The knowledge of old theories offers an additional advantage to the doctor in that many of his patients still cling to a variety of medical beliefs which can be traced to the Stone Age, the ancient Greeks, Paracelsus, or the Scotsman John Brown. Of course, even more important, but also far more difficult to know, is what doctors did in the past. Theory and practice sometimes differ considerably.

Medical history is more than "mental gymnastics." The history of clinical observation and therapeutics, and particularly of the diseases, furnishes data which, if properly handled, will still yield new insights. But even if medical history lacked these immediately useful aspects, it would be far from valueless. Scientific medicine became possible only through cultivation of the not immediately useful. The rapid rise of medicine in this country in recent years coincides very closely with the large-scale introduction into the medical curriculum of what is not immediately useful. The "useful" detail, on the other hand, is often quickly superseded and has to be dropped.

It must also be emphasized that disease is more than the physiological and psychological breakdown of an individual. Powerful social factors determine whether people fall sick or not, and how and with what results they are treated. A doctor cannot appreciate too early the fact that his profession is a part and product of society and that it is always closely connected with religion, philosophy, economics, politics, and the whole of human culture. His education, social status, and remuneration—and, unfortunately, his specialization as well—depend in the last instance on the tastes and decisions of society. Medical history is forced to deal with this nonscientific social background of medicine and thus serves, as no other medical discipline can, to open the eyes to those social factors without which the problems of health and disease cannot be properly understood.

Medicine is not only a science; it is also an art. Science is primarily analytic, art primarily synthetic. Medicine is likely to remain an art, however hard we may try to make it more and more scientific, and however much we may attempt to master its scientific contents. For medicine deals not with impersonal atoms, elements, plants with tropisms, or animals with instinct mechanisms, but with humans with a "soul" and "free will." In order to fulfill his mission, therefore, the physician has to be more than a mere technician and man of science. He must be a well-rounded human being, humane and humanistic. In practice he deals not with disordered metabolisms, specific infections, or neoplasms, but with sick human individuals. Even the effect of digitalis or antibiotics will partially depend on the human relationship between the doctor and his patient, not to speak of treatment of the "psychosomatic" diseases that will normally form from 50 to 70 per cent of the doctor's practice.

Science so far has contributed little to this aspect of the doctor's work. In fact, technical education has pulled in the opposite direction. It has let its experience with laboratory animals color too deeply its outlook on man. It has offered the abstractions of science as a substitute for a knowledge of human nature. It is true that knowledge can be picked up in the trial-and-error method of daily practice, but that is a long and costly way of learning. Medical history can at least help shorten the period of trial and error by showing medicine in perspective, as a colorful product of man in all his strength and weakness. Even the pitifully small fragments of general knowledge of human history and behavior which are transmitted in medicohistorical teaching may sometimes help in nurturing and developing the deeper understanding of human nature so badly needed by the physician.

Medical education is complete only if it implants certain moral and ethical values in the future doctor. The doctor after all is human too, entitled to a decent living for his family and himself, and forced to find a sound balance between sacrifice and legitimate self-interest in the exercise of his profession. The pressures and temptations to lower his standards for the sake of money and popularity are numerous. Here again medical history can play a valuable role, second perhaps only to the personal example of the medical teacher. Those acquainted with the teachings of Hippocrates, with the lives of such men as Paré, Lister, Pasteur, or Osler, will find in them ever-flowing sources of moral strength.

A man can be a competent doctor without a knowledge of medical history. But an acquaintance with medical history can make him a better doctor. It is no accident that so many of the great doctors of the last hundred years, whether the name be Osler, Halsted, Welch, Cushing, Andral, Virchow, Wunderlich, Claude Bernard, Charcot, Pasteur, Sherrington, Zinsser, Richet, Löffler, Behring, or Sauerbruch, have had a profound interest in medical history and have often made valuable contributions to the field.

While the study of medical history can be rewarding to everybody, no one will profit more from it than the medical student. It can considerably shorten the period of trial and error, so painful to him—and to his patients. Medical history will show him, long before he could discover for himself in his own professional life, how drugs and gadgets come and go, how often it is suggestion that actually produces the cure, how soon the useful detail of today is superseded by a better one, and how sometimes even positive acquisitions have grown out of irrational approaches, half-truths, and sheer empiricism. Anyone who has seen how the truth of today becomes the error of tomorrow will adopt a more independent and critical attitude and will be better equipped to assimilate new truths. This is of prime importance, for many members of the medical profession have at all times displayed a queer mixture of unreasonable conservatism and no more reasonable addiction to the latest novelties. Only those who have followed the slow and painful growth of the art and science of medicine, only those who know how much has been accomplished and how much still remains to be done, only those who know how many centuries and even millennia it took to build up knowledge which is now taken for granted, can see this science in its proper proportion, can feel appropriate pride in the medical profession, supposedly the oldest profession of all, and can acquire the humility so necessary to all humans, laymen and doctors.

A SHORT HISTORY OF MEDICINE

Chapter 1

PALEOPATHOLOGY AND PALEOMEDICINE

The earliest documents on medical history, the Egyptian papyri, carry the story back only about four thousand years. Nevertheless, there are methods which allow us at least a notion of what was going on during the millions of years before the invention of writing. These are the methods of the prehistorian and the paleontologist, which can be put to use by medical historians who want to know something about the beginnings of disease and its treatments. The medical historian can study teeth and bones (often fossilized), mummies, and prehistoric works of art. He can also take account of the immunological behavior of infectious diseases, which gives some idea of their age and origin. These methods are, of course, extremely fragmentary. Changes in bones will tell us nothing about the numerous diseases limited to the soft tissues and organs. Only a very small number of bones survive the accidents of erosion and the practice of cremation which was common in so many early societies. Many of the bone changes admit several interpretations. The science dealing with this paleontological and prehistoric evidence of disease is called *paleopathology*.

Problematic as these materials may be, they all tell the same story. In spite of the legend of a golden, happy, diseaseless age in the remote past—a legend cherished in almost all cultures—disease is very old, far older than mankind, in fact almost as old as life on earth. Our evidence also tells us that disease forms have remained essentially the same throughout the millions of years.

3

Fossilized bacteria similar to our present-day micrococci can be found in geological formations that are 500,000,000 years old. Whether these bacteria were pathogenic is, of course, impossible to decide. Charles Nicolle suggested that the oldest pathogenic bacteria were of the gram-positive type with spores. (Gram-positive bacteria are so called because they retain dye when treated after the method of Gram.) Next in age he placed the gram-positive bacteria without spores and the gram-negative bacteria. He regarded viruses as the youngest of the pathogenic organisms because of their advanced parasitism and specialization.

Fossil shells of 350,000,000 years ago reveal that parasitism and traumatism were disturbing living animal forms at that early date. The ailments of the great reptiles of 200,000,000 years ago can be established from the evidence of surviving bones. The dinosaurs, mososaurs, and crocodiles of the period frequently experienced fractures, and many of these fractures healed more or less well. In spite of not being addicted to the consumption of alcohol and tobacco or the dietary errors of civilization, these reptiles show frequent signs of chronic arthritis, one of the main problems of present-day medical practice. Inflammatory processes of the bone, such as osteo-myelitis and osteoperiostitis, are observed, as well as benign tumors (osteoma, hemangioma) and dental caries.

Many of the fossilized reptiles are found in a position of opisthotonos (overextension of the vertebral column). Since opisthotonos is a sign of inflammation of the meninges of the brain, the hypothesis is not unwarranted that such animals died from infectious diseases affecting these organs.

Sixty million years ago the mammals became dominant. The pathology of fossil mammals is essentially the same as that observed in the big reptiles; here again are found frac-tures, osteoarthritis, infectious bone diseases, tumors, etc. The bones of cave bears of the Pleistocene epoch, which were among the first pathological bones studied, showed striking evidence of arthritis. As a result, this disease as displayed in prehistoric animals has been called cave gout. This is undoubtedly a misnomer, since osteoarthritis is also found in humans and animals that live, not in humid caves, but in the driest and hottest regions of the earth. The German patholo- gist Virchow, who was one of the first to describe this "cave gout" in bears, rightly emphasized the fact that some of their tibiae showed the changes usually regarded as evidence of syphilis when found in the bones of pre-Columbian American Indians.

In view of the fact that most of the prehistoric species fell victims to extinction, it is pertinent to ask whether disease, rather than change of climate or other unknown factors, may not have been the cause of their disappearance. The bone dis- eases observed and described so far do not warrant such a conclusion. These chronic diseases may have been painful and troublesome, but they were not fatal. On the other hand, diseases of other types may in some cases have had something to do with the extinction of animal species. This is suggested by the occurrence of fossilized flies of the "tsetse" type in the American Tertiary. The tsetse fly is today the transmitter of trypanosomiasis, the deadly parasitic infection which afflicts man and cattle in Africa.

A large incidence of disease is compatible with survival. This apparent contradiction of the beliefs of Darwin is sup- ported by studies of contemporary wild animals. Particularly impressive in this respect are the studies of Adolph Schultz, who killed and dissected a whole colony of gibbons in Malaysia. He not only found a very high percentage of frac- tures (many well healed), arthritis, and osteitis in these apes, but also discovered that 90 per cent of them were suffering from filariasis, 10 per cent from malaria, and 40 per cent from some kind of trypanosomiasis. In addition he found caries, sinusitis, hernia, cryptorchism (undescended testicles), and spina bifida. In view of the relationship between man and gibbon, a similar infestation of man's ancestors seems rather likely.

Man seems to have been a ready victim of disease ever since he began to emerge from Simian darkness some 500,000 years ago. Dubois' *Pithecanthropus*, excavated in Java in 1891, and for decades the oldest known early human specimen, shows a great exostosis (morbid bony growth) on his femur. The next oldest group of early men, the Neanderthal, found everywhere in Europe, Africa, and the Near East, shows clear evidence of arthritis and traumatism followed by suppuration. The enormously fat females represented in the earliest works of Paleolithic art (about 25,000 B.C.), and ironically called "Venuses," may also have been pathological specimens.

While modern man roamed in Neolithic Europe (about 10,000 B.C.) he suffered, again according to his bones, from traumatism, arthritis, sinusitis, tumors, spina bifida, and congenital dislocation of the hip. One Neolithic skeleton found in Germany also showed evidence of tuberculosis of the vertebral column (Pott's disease). Problematic cases of rickets have been found in Scandinavia and problematic sequels of poliomyelitis in Neolithic England.

The richest documentation on paleopathology undoubtedly stems from Egypt, where it has been possible to study mummies in addition to bone material. Through the ceaseless energy of men like Armand Ruffer, Grafton Elliot Smith, and Wood Jones, the remnants of no less than 36,000 individuals have been examined. The bone records tell the familiar story. Arthritis is indicated in skeletons dating back to 4000 B.C. One skeleton (3400 B.C.) suggests the existence of poliomyelitis, and others reveal tuberculosis of the hip joint (2700 B.C.) and of the vertebral column (2000 B.C.). Many fractures are found, often well healed, and there is frequent testimony to the existence of inflammatory processes (mastoiditis), tumors (osteoma and osteosarcoma), and club foot. This bone evidence is confirmed by the art of this period, which portrays persons suffering from the sequels of poliomyelitis, from club foot, from Pott's disease, and from achondroplastic dwarfism. No signs of syphilis or rickets are found in these Egyptian bones. Malignant bone tumors are seen in skulls from the fourth and third millennium B.C. On the other hand, osteoporosis (brittleness) of the skull, a very rare condition among modern Europeans, is found rather frequently.

The examination of the tissues of mummies enlarges our horizons considerably and makes strikingly clear how little can be discovered about the pathology of the past through the study of bones alone. In these mummies highly developed arteriosclerosis has been found, as well as pneumonia, pleurisy, kidney stones, gallstones, and appendicitis. Schistosomiasis, still a prevalent disease in Egypt, has been noted in kidneys three thousand years old. Skin lesions in some mummies suggest smallpox (1100 B.C.), a disease otherwise described first in the Middle Ages. Prolapsus of the uterus and intestines, and sequels of birth accidents, have also been found in Egyptian mummies.

The situation in the Americas is much the same. It is among the Peruvian Indians that the richest collections of remains are found. These show evidence of arthritis, sinusitis, bone tumors (osteosarcoma and multiple myeloma), and osteoporosis. After the recent discoveries of Antonio Requena and W. Ritchie, it seems beyond doubt that pre-Columbian Indians suffered from tuberculosis of the vertebral column. A number of pre-Columbian American forms have been said to exhibit syphilitic changes. The existence of syphilis in the Old World before the discovery of America has also been claimed on the basis of paleopathological evidence. But it seems wiser, and more in accordance with the facts, to say only that the bones show remnants of an osteitis of unknown origin. Present techniques do not allow more positive conclusions.

Peruvian mummies, like those in Egypt, show arteriosclerotic changes. Mummies of the "Basketmakers," a prehistoric North American Indian culture, show signs of bronchopneumonia and silicosis. In spite of its ubiquity, arthritis shows differences of localization in different genera, species, races, and civilizations. The fact that diseases vary from civilization to civilization makes paleopathological materials valuable for the study of societies as well as individuals.

So much for the pathology of ancient man. But when it comes to the question of the *medicine* of these men, it must be confessed that the evidence is more than scanty. Many findings, formerly interpreted as expressions of paleomedicine ("paleomedicine" is used here to denote the medicine of ancient man, as opposed to "primitive medicine," the medicine of contemporary savages), have been shown to have no medical significance. For instance, the finger amputations depicted on the walls of caverns are probably of a religious nature. The so-called *batons de commande* (scepters), which were once thought to be the paraphernalia of prehistoric medicine men, have been observed to fulfill the more prosaic role of arrow sharpeners among contemporary Eskimos. Nor does the occurrence of well-healed fractures in prehistoric bones prove the existence of experienced bonesetters. This is the unavoidable conclusion to be drawn from Adolph Schultz' gibbon material, which is so rich in such pieces. There remains only one substantial piece of evidence of prehistoric medical activity. Trephined skulls are found all over Europe in Neolithic deposits. They are also to be found in Peru, where the earliest is perhaps two thousand years old. When the first of such skulls were found and described in the eighteen seventies, it seemed hard to believe that primitive man had been able to carry through successfully, with simple stone knives, an operation then greatly dreaded by contemporary surgeons. Some of the so-called trepanations could be discarded as malformations, traumatisms, or artifacts. Yet the ever-increasing bulk of the material, combined with the observation of the same operation among contemporary primitives, made the conclusion unavoidable that Neolithic man actually did trephine successfully on a rather large scale.

Still to be settled is the meaning of this daring operation for our Stone Age predecessors. The great French surgeon and anthropologist, Paul Broca, who was the first to study the trephined skulls and the operation techniques involved, was inclined to derive the practice primarily from belief in supernaturalistic theories of disease. He felt that primitive

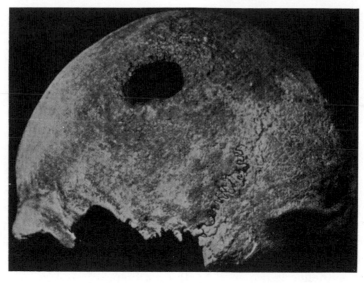

Figure 1. Trephined neolithic skull.

man had made these holes in the skull in order to liberate evil spirits who might be causing headaches or epilepsy. Fortifying him in this assumption was the fact that the bone disks, or rondelles, excised in the operation were used as amulets. Broca's explanation was challenged by later students who held that the operation was of an entirely practical and rational nature. The Austrian anthropologist D. Woelfel observed that trepanations were practiced most widely in areas where weapons producing skull fractures were used. He felt that the operation was introduced in order to remove bone fragments and relieve intracranial pressure in the case of head wounds. The hope of finding a solution to the problem in the observation of contemporary trephining among primitives has not been fulfilled. Both forms of practice, the supernaturalistic and the naturalistic, have been observed. But it is important to note that the operation of trepanation has remained an entirely isolated accomplishment among those primitives who practice it; in other ways they are extremely poor surgeons. Also, the practice has been kept a strict secret by the tribes of the Andean highlands. These facts are in favor of Broca's old supernaturalistic hypothesis.

Chapter 2

PRIMITIVE MEDICINE

Direct evidence on the medicine of early man is, as we have seen, extremely meager. There is, however, some indirect evidence which, when used cautiously and with full awareness of its problematic character, can give valuable hints about the character of the medicine of the dim past. This evidence is provided by the medicine of contemporary savages or primitives—so-called primitive medicine. It must be used cautiously, since none of these tribes can portray medical practices exactly as they were carried out seven or eight thousand years ago. It is true that these primitive societies have remained fundamentally on a Stone Age level. But the fact that they have not developed to more advanced levels in technology, social organization, and ideology does not mean that they have remained static. Though these tribes do not have a written history, they have been subject to historical change, just as have the civilizations from which our own culture emerged. But the rate of change in primitive societies is markedly slower than in more dynamic civilizations. Thus it is reasonable to assume that they have maintained many characteristics of their prehistoric predecessors, in the field of medicine as in other fields.

The study of primitive medicine would be fruitful and informative if it were undertaken solely with the object of gaining these historical insights. But there is an even more important reason for studying it. The fascinating feature of primitive medicine is that it represents a medical system utterly different from our own, yet one that functions satisfactorily. It is primarily with this functional point of view in mind that primitive medicine will be analyzed here.

The best way to become familiar with primitive medicine is to observe a typical medical treatment as it is actually carried through in a given contemporary primitive society. An Apache feels ill. He and his family behave much as would the modern man. At first there is not much speculation as to the character and origin of his "indisposition." The patient rests, and household remedies are applied. Only when no improvement can be obtained in this way does the sick man really think of "disease." It is here that the ways of the two types of medicine separate. The sick Apache assumes that his disease has been caused by a supernatural agency such as an animal spirit, a ghost, or a sorcerer. Accordingly he summons, not a scientific doctor, but a magician, the medicine man. Not just any medicine man will do. He takes some care to call a specialist—the medicine man who is known to have particular supernatural powers against the particular agency which the patient suspects to be at the bottom of his trouble.

The medicine man, the family, and the friends of the patient gather round his bed and start a ceremony which lasts for four days and nights. The ceremony consists of prayers and magic formulas, of drumming, and of touching the patient with such sacred objects as pollens, feathers, and turquoise. The medicine man tries to obtain a kind of anamnesis by making the patient recall his past and confess possible offenses against the religious or social rules of his tribe. Then the guardian spirit or "power" of the medicine man "reveals" to him the cause, the prognosis, and the necessary treatment of the disease. If the Apache has been the victim of a sorcerer, the medicine man "sucks out" disease-producing "arrows," such as small bones or pebbles, from the body of the patient. In other cases the treatment is simpler. Drugs are prescribed; the patient is given a magic amulet; and perhaps he is forbidden to have a shadow fall upon him or to eat certain foods; that is, a taboo is imposed.

Similar ideas concerning the causes of disease will be found in all primitive societies. They are called magico-religious or supernaturalistic ideas. All primitives will assume that the majority of diseases are sent by ghosts, spirits, or gods offended by some taboo violation. In other cases the disease may be thought to have been inflicted by a sorcerer, a mortal in control of supernatural forces. Such a man may have been hired to send the disease, or he may simply send it because he has been offended in some way by the patient or his family.

The supernatural forces bring about disease by shooting foreign matter into the body of the patient or by introducing spirits into it. This explains the fear of injections exhibited by many primitives. Other primitives believe in the existence of several souls in one body and assume that disease is caused by abduction of one of these souls from the sufferer. Supernaturalistic beliefs concerning the cause of disease have by no means died out in the less-educated strata of the American people and in remote districts of other civilized countries. If a patient attributes his disease to sorcery, it is not always safe to assume that he suffers from paranoia. He may only be proffering what in his milieu is still a legitimate explanation of disease.

It is only logical that diseases caused by supernatural agencies can be diagnosed only by supernatural techniques. Therefore, diagnostics in primitive society consist primarily of the application of one of the many divination procedures invented by man in the course of history. The procedure chosen may be crystal gazing, bone throwing (a predecessor of card playing, which was originally a divinatory procedure), or a trance entered into by the medicine man.

Treatment, too, has to be primarily of a supernaturalistic nature. Invisible disease-producing foreign bodies have to be sucked out or removed by dry cupping. This mechanical procedure has to be reinforced by magic spells or by the application of medicines, internal or external, which are thought to be effective because of their magic power. Happily, some of these drugs do in fact produce beneficial effects. Intruding spirits have to be driven out by magico-religious formulas, by noise, sometimes even by beating the patient, and, last but not least, by bloodletting. The abducted soul has to be hunted by the soul of the medicine man, who has the power to separate himself from his own soul in a state of trance. In the case of the taboo violation, the guardian spirits have to be pacified by confession—which is of a psychological value in itself—by sacrifices, or by purification ceremonies such as artificially induced vomiting, purging, baths, or a special diet. All therapeutic measures, objective and subjective, are elements of a magico-religious ritual centered around the spell. It is no accident that the oldest documents in Germanic are the Merseburg spells against bleeding and fractures in men and animals.

Because of its supernaturalistic character, primitive prophylaxis has often been left unrecognized. Yet there is no doubt that amulets, ritual mutilations such as circumcision, and the ritual painting of the body are all measures designed to prevent disease. Ritual scarification sometimes includes real inoculation against smallpox or snakebite. Primitives usually do away with their excrements in a sanitary way, although their reasons are by no means identical with those of modern times. The hiding of excrements is induced by the fear that such material could be appropriated by sorcerers who might use it against the original owner by casting a spell on it. Clipped nails, cut hair, and other separated parts of the body are also used for such spells.

A supernatural orientation is the fundamental trait of primitive medicine and is the main ground for the basic differences between the primitive medical approach and modern scientific methods. The fact that during a greater part of its existence humanity has believed in supernatural forces, rather than in natural law, makes the study of primitive medicine, weird as it may seem to the contemporary observer, not just an excusable pastime but an imperative need.

If one wonders why primitives resort to these unrealistic, supernaturalistic explanations and measures, one should realize that disease is for them, even more than for us, a problem of the very greatest urgency. Under this pressure they resort to an explanation that seems to them the most plausible. For man who, unlike the animal, remains dependent for years after his birth—a peculiarity already known to Locke and Rousseau—this explanation is not nature but the family or society. A fictitious, supernatural family of totemic animals, ghosts, or gods sends diseases arbitrarily, or as a punishment for violating social rules. Disease thus becomes invested with a meaning it does not possess with us.

The consequences of supernaturalist beliefs can be observed in all branches of medicine. The anatomical knowledge of primitives, for instance, is notoriously poor, in spite of the fact that some of them open a great number of human and animal bodies. Anatomical knowledge cannot be acquired by people who are not primarily interested in natural causes in connection with disease. This is illustrated by the fact that even in those primitive tribes which perform autopsies—they open bodies regularly in order to detect "witchcraft principles"—anatomical knowledge is as poor as among those who perform no such autopsies.

The supernaturalistic approach goes far toward explaining the strange contradictions of primitive surgery. Tribes that in other respects have developed no surgical techniques more complicated than their neighbors are often able to perform a few very complicated operations, such as trephining, cesarean section, and subincision of the penis. The fact that people who have invented such complicated operations, and carried them through successfully, should not develop any other active surgery can be understood only if it is assumed that such operations grow primarily out of supernatural rather than technical considerations. It is equally hard to understand why people who amputate or mutilate extensively for religious or judiciary reasons do not carry over those operations into the field of medicine, amputating, for example, a hopelessly infected and mangled limb. Such behavior can be explained only by the fact that their "surgery" remains for them in the supernaturalistic sphere.

Primitive pharmacopeias present a strange mixture of innumerable ineffective drugs with a few of marked effect which are valued elements of our own pharmacopeia. This fact can be understood only when it is realized that primitives approach their drugs, not from the point of view of empirical checking for effectiveness, but from the point of view of magic power and magic relations.

Primitive medicine is spared the conflicts which in modern times have called psychosomatic medicine into being. Primitives do not in general make a distinction between organic, functional, and mental diseases. For them there is only disease and its treatment, a treatment which always contains psychotherapeutic as well as objective elements. This holistic or unitary character is one of the outstanding traits of primitive medicine. Diagnostics is at the same time therapeutics, organic treatment is used in mental disease, and the mental approach is applied to organic disease.

To modern man disease is a biological phenomenon that concerns him only as an individual and has no moral implications. When he contracts influenza or tuberculosis, he never attributes this event to his behavior toward the tax collector or his mother-in-law. Among primitives, because of their supernaturalistic theories, the prevailing moral point of view gives a deeper meaning to disease. The gods and sorcerers who send disease are usually angered by the moral trespasses of the individual. Sometimes they may not strike the guilty person himself, but rather one of his relatives or tribesmen, to whom responsibility is extended. Disease, action that might produce disease, and reparation of disease are, therefore, of vital concern to the whole primitive community. Disease, as a sanction against social misbehavior, becomes one of the most important pillars of order in such societies. It takes over, in many cases, the role played by policemen, judges, and priests in modern society. In primitive societies, biological or psychological abnormalities offer only the occasion to diagnose a disease. Whether this is eventually done depends on the decisions of society. There are societies where intestinal worms, umbilical hernias, malaria, yaws, or certain dermatoses are not regarded as diseases.

The study of primitive medicine has a practical value quite apart from the general considerations suggested above. Such stand-bys of modern practice as the drugs picrotoxin, emetine, strophanthin, serpasil, and cocaine were all derived from primitive pharmacopeias. No doubt others of equal value remain to be discovered. And it is probable that modern medicine has added little to the fundamental psychotherapeutic mechanisms unconsciously used by the medicine man—confession and suggestion.

The medicine man was on the whole successful. His success was probably due to the social and psychotherapeutical mechanisms described, to a few effective drugs, and to effective physical therapy methods such as massage and bathing. It is important to remember, too, the kind of diseases with which he had to deal. The epidemic diseases—typhoid, measles, diphtheria, smallpox, yellow fever, and cholera—which have constituted one of the main problems of recent medicine, were unknown to primitives before the arrival of the white man. Chronic infections had reached a certain equilibrium. Degenerative diseases and cancer were equally rare in a population whose life expectancy was low because of the infant and accident mortality. The medicine man was primarily faced by rheumatic diseases, digestive disturbances, respiratory diseases, skin diseases, gynecological disorders, and the whole gamut of functional disturbances. To deal with these he was rather well equipped.

The medicine man has often been accused of being either a fake or a psychopath. The former accusation was based mainly on his practice of sucking out disease-producing stones; the latter was derived from his trances. Anthropological research of the last fifty years has shown that the average medicine man is just as sincere as the modern doctor. If he contracts disease himself, he willingly undergoes treatment by another medicine man. His famous stone-sucking ritual has to be understood as one of those symbolic actions found in all religious rites. Trance, which existed in our own society until a few hundred years ago, cannot be regarded as psychopathological in societies in which it is developed as a normal religious experience. A person of the social rank and integration of the medicine man is not likely to be a psychopath, that is, a maladjusted individual. As a matter of fact, even those medicine men who do undergo a psychosis in their preparatory period, such as the Siberian and South African shamans, are demonstrably well balanced after they have actually reached the stage of shamanistic practice.

The field of interest of the medicine man is both more generalized and more specialized than that of the present-day doctor. Being a magician, the medicine man does not limit the exercise of his magic power exclusively to fighting against disease but is also likely to practice magic in such spheres as war, love, and hunting. He is specialized in the sense that he usually possesses magic formulas to combat only a few diseases —sometimes only one. This is a specialization which stems from too little knowledge rather than too much. Since magic formulas are either acquired by inheritance, bought for a heavy price from a teacher, or revealed in visions, it is obvious that the medicine man in general can have only a few of these precious spells in his possession. Specialization also runs along functional lines. There are herbalists, bonesetters, and medicine men proper (physicians). But none of these sub-groups of medical personnel among primitives—not even the midwives—is ever free from the all-pervading supernaturalistic orientation.

The above statements are of course abstractions. In any given primitive society, only some of the phenomena described above will be found, and they will seldom fall into the same patterns. It depends on the total context of a given culture whether medical rites will play an important role or be insignificant, whether emotional or empirical elements will be in the foreground, whether medicine men are highly trained specialists or plain tribesmen engaged in curing as a side line. One of the most surprising results of modern anthropological research is the discovery that even the notion of the abnormal may change from one culture to another. Thus a biological phenomenon which is considered normal in one culture may be regarded as abnormal and pathological in another.

Chapter 3

MEDICINE OF ANCIENT CIVILIZATIONS

In a few places favored by nature, in the great river valleys of the Old World and on the high plateaus of the New World, tribal groups grew into empires and developed urban civilizations. The inhabitants of these empires developed writing. Information concerning them can be derived from written records as well as from rich archeological findings. At this point history proper begins.

It is obvious that the large general changes in social structure, technology, and ideology incurred in the development of empires also brought about important changes in medicine. Within the limits of this book the general background cannot be discussed. Only their medicine can be considered, and even then it is necessary to limit this account to the outstanding civilizations—ancient Egypt, Babylonia, Mexico, and Peru. Space will not allow discussion of the ancient Persians, Jews, Phoenicians, Cretans, and Etruscans.

Social change influenced pathology as well as medicine. Only the densely settled empires and their large cities made it possible for the acute infections to last and for the great epidemics to spread. They began to dominate the pathological picture and did so until the twentieth century.

❉   ❉   ❉

Egyptian medicine enjoyed great fame in antiquity. Homer (about 1000 B.C.) speaks of the Egyptians as being the best doctors. Herodotus in the fifth century B.C. comments enthusiastically on Egyptian physicians and speaks of the

19

population of Egypt as being particularly healthy, in striking contrast to what was observed in the Middle Ages and modern times. Inscriptions dating as far back as the Fifth Dynasty (2700 B.C.) prove the existence of physicians and dentists in Egypt, especially at court. Some even bore such poetic titles as "Shepherd of the Anus." The anus was the main seat of pathology, while the heart was the center of life. Egyptian physicians were in demand in all the courts of the Near East before the advent of Greek physicians.

In spite of the existence of a special medical profession in Egypt, supernaturalism, especially in the form of religion, remained dominant in the realm of disease and its treatment. This is not surprising in a civilization whose king was a god, whose pyramids and mummies bore witness to its tremendous preoccupation with life after death, and whose priests played an important political role. Physicians were trained in temple schools and probably remained priests all their lives in the manner of later medieval priest-physicians in the West. Spirits and demons continued to "cause" diseases, and spells continued to be used against them. But spells tended to be replaced more and more by prayers, and demons were overshadowed by gods. Special gods gave protection against special diseases and invented new remedies for them, while other gods were the authors of disease. Sometimes the same god would both send a disease and cure it. Each limb of the body was connected with a special god—to such an extent that Sigerist can speak appropriately of the "mythological anatomy" of the Egyptians. Amulets were used extensively. Re, Thoth, and Isis were important healing gods. Sekhmet, the Lady of Pestilence, brought on epidemics and removed them.

In the last centuries of Egyptian civilization all the gods were overshadowed by a new healing god, Imhotep. Imhotep is a historical figure, Vizier of a Pharaoh who lived about 2900 B.C. His name means "the one who walked in peace." He is credited with many accomplishments in many fields, and one of his activities seems to have been that of

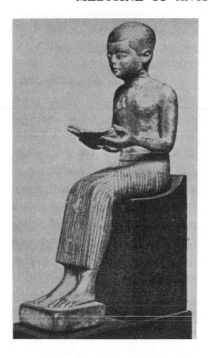

FIGURE 2. Imhotep, the Egyptian
god of medicine.

a successful physician. He is thus one of the first medical
men whose name is on record, and, like the later Asclepius,
he rose from the role of medical hero to become God of
Medicine. Like Asclepius he cured by "incubation," i.e.,
during sleep in his temple. But, in spite of this general
supernaturalistic orientation, the highly organized medicine
of Egypt is found to contain an impressive amount of empiricism such as is quite unknown to primitive societies.
Here is the beginning of a rational theory of disease and life
in general.

Our knowledge of Egyptian medicine is based on certain
papyri, books written on material made from stems of the
papyrus plant. Because of the perishable nature of this material, only a handful of books concerning medical practice
have been preserved. The most recent papyrus reflects the
medical ideas of about three thousand years ago, and most of
the books probably pertain to a considerably older period,

perhaps five or six thousand years ago. Naturally any generalization covering a span of more than two thousand years and based on such meager evidence must be of a hypothetical nature.

The oldest known medical papyrus, the so-called *Kahun Papyrus** (about 2000 B.C.), deals with gynecology and veterinary medicine. The two most important papyri are the *Edwin Smith Papyrus* (about 1600 B.C.), dealing with surgery, and the *Ebers Papyrus* (about 1550 B.C.), a kind of medical textbook. The great *Berlin Papyrus* (1300 B.C.) and the *Hearst Papyrus* (1500 B.C.) are very similar to the *Ebers Papyrus*. However, their contents are largely restricted to prescriptions, and they contain more magical elements than the *Ebers Papyrus*. The *London Papyrus* (1350 B.C.) is purely magical in tone. And the same holds true for the lesser Berlin papyrus (*Westcar*), and the Berlin papyrus No. 3027 (*Brugsch Minor*), dealing with obstetrics.

The fact that the more recent papyri are far more magical in content than the older ones has led to the belief that Egyptian medicine started out with a comparatively rational approach and became more and more magical with the decline of Egyptian civilization. Such a development is perfectly possible, as is made clear by the examples of late antiquity and the Middle Ages in Europe. But the evidence is too scanty to make such a conclusion certain. There may have been a strong magical element in early Egyptian medicine of which we remain ignorant because fate preserved only the more empirical writings. And for later periods the empirical writings could have been lost and only the magical ones preserved.

Most informative of these writings are the *Edwin Smith Papyrus* and the *Ebers Papyrus*. They both reveal considerable talent in presenting case histories and in establishing a generalized disease notion. In both papyri the case approach is as follows: (1) the provisory diagnosis; (2) instructions on

---

* Egyptologists name a papyrus either after the man who first acquired it or after the place where the manuscript is kept.

how to examine the patient and the diagnostic signs to be looked for; (3) the diagnosis and prognosis of the case; and (4) an indication of the necessary therapeutic measures, such as manipulation, drugs, and magic formulas or prayers. This scheme can be clearly seen in the following case described in the *Edwin Smith Papyrus:*

Instructions concerning a dislocation of a vertebra of his neck: If you examine a man having a dislocation of a vertebra of his neck, should you find him unconscious of his arms and legs on account of it, while his phallus is erected on account of it and sperm drops from his member without his knowing; his flesh has received wind; his eyes are bloodshot—then you should say concerning him: He has a dislocation of a vertebra of his neck, since he is unconscious of his legs and arms, and his sperm dribbles. An ailment which cannot be treated.[1]

The same thoroughness in diagnosis is illustrated in the following case recorded in the *Ebers Papyrus:*

If thou examinest a man for an illness in his cardia, and all his limbs are heavy for him as [at] an access of debility, then thou shalt put thy hand over his cardia; if thou findest his cardia drumming [i.e., tympanitic] and it is going and coming under thy fingers, then thou shalt say about it: it is a weakness of digestion that has prevented him from eating before. Thou shalt effect all his evacuation for him: njt of dates, is pulped with beer nt 'k, then gets his appetite. If thou examinest him after this has been done, and thou findest his breast-side warm and his belly cool, then thou shalt say: his weakness [of digestion] has gone down [i.e., is healed]. Thou shalt let him guard his mouth against all *d3f.*[2]

The *Edwin Smith Papyrus* is a fragment consisting of forty-eight cases, mainly head injuries. The cases are arranged according to a pattern observed by medical writers up to the end of the eighteenth century, *a capite ad calcem* (from the head down to the feet). A high level of clinical observation is revealed in the descriptions of such phenomena as the feeble pulse, palsy, and deafness resulting from

---

[1] J. H. Breasted (ed.), *Edwin Smith Surgical Papyrus* (Chicago, 1930), Vol. I, p. 324.

[2] *Ebers Papyrus,* trans. by Ebbell (Copenhagen, 1937), p. 47.

head injuries. The papyrus is unfortunately incomplete and ends at the level of the thorax. Although this is a surgical papyrus, use of the knife, today considered the essence of surgery, is not mentioned. Neither here nor elsewhere is any evidence of trephining in ancient Egypt found. The only "source" of this rumor is a popular novel and the movie made from it. This is a reminder of the fact that the surgeon of the past limited himself to wound treatment and bonesetting, and that operative procedures remained rare in the average surgeon's practice up to the second half of the nineteenth century. Stitching, splints, and the use of the fire drill are mentioned. In the magic vein the papyrus contains incantations against pestilential winds and for rejuvenation. Here for the first time is encountered the refusal of the medical practitioner to treat hopeless cases, an attitude which remained legitimate and ethical with many as late as the eighteenth century.

The *Ebers Papyrus* is a kind of medical textbook. It starts out with three incantations to be used in giving remedies or loosening bandages. There follow books on internal diseases; eye diseases, which seem to have plagued the ancient Egyptians just as they do their modern descendants; skin diseases; diseases of the extremities; miscellaneous diseases; and women's diseases. An eighth book deals with anatomy and physiology, and the ninth and last book is devoted to surgery. Here surgery is a little more active than in the *Edwin Smith Papyrus*. The numerous names for diseases and organs, the attempts to use all available senses for diagnostic purposes, and the construction of disease entities on the basis of clinical symptoms, all testify to the relatively high development of medicine in the period of the *Ebers Papyrus*. The pathological conditions described in the papyrus, such as rheumatism and schistosomiasis, have also been revealed to some extent in the examination of the mummies of the period. A condition resembling diabetes is described. A leading role is played by the different diseases caused by worms: hookworm, filaria, taenia, and ascaris. This may explain why the

Egyptians interpreted so many diseases by means of a theory of invasion by worms. The papyrus contains 876 prescriptions made up from more than five hundred substances. These include such minerals as lead and copper salts, vegetable matter such as gentian, senna, castor oil seed, pomegranate as vermifuge, scilla, henbane, and animal substances. Raw liver was prescribed against night blindness. The prescriptions tend to be composed of numerous substances (polypharmacy), and they contain not a little of the *Dreckapotheke*—urine and excrements of man or animals. It is surprising that neither diet nor venesection is mentioned.

Recognition of the clinical acumen of the *Edwin Smith Papyrus* and the *Ebers Papyrus* should not blind the reader to the very substantial evidence of supernaturalism in Egyptian medicine. Magic formulas, amulets, and exorcisms are mentioned in these books. The fact that cleanliness and hygiene are emphasized in the papyri, as well as in the whole Egyptian culture, is no proof whatsoever for the absence of supernaturalism. On the contrary, cleanliness, which even with us is next to godliness, seems often to have definite religious roots. In earlier societies people seem to have kept clean, not primarily for practical reasons, but in order to be pure in the eyes of the gods. A positive correlation between holiness and dirt has been established in only a few societies.

Egyptian anatomy as reflected in the *Ebers Papyrus*, though rational in spirit, is mainly speculative. It is interesting to note that this nation of embalmers acquired no positive knowledge of anatomy. Anatomy and physiology seem to have been based on the existence of the heart, forty-four (or twenty-two) hypothetical vessels, and the life-giving role of the breath. The appreciation of vessels is not surprising in a country whose existence depended on irrigation canals. The Egyptians appear to have developed the notion of the fundamental four elements—earth, water, fire, and air—that played such an important role in medicine up to modern times.

Herodotus mentions extreme specialization as one of the outstanding characteristics of Egyptian medicine. In view of the fact that the earliest extant document on Egyptian medicine is a specialist's document, it is a tenable presumption that specialization in Egyptian medicine was not an end product, but rather a carry-over from primitive specialization. Thus such compilations as the *Ebers Papyrus* would represent a later praiseworthy attempt to overcome primitive specialization.

Rigid traditionalism was, again according to Herodotus, an outstanding characteristic of Egyptian medicine, a view which is supported by what is known of the total attitude of Egyptian civilization. Three types of healing personnel are mentioned in Egyptian documents: physicians, exorcists, and "priests of Sekhmet," who have been regarded as surgeons or as specialists in feeling the pulse and treating diseases of the vessels. Most is known, of course, about the court physicians, who were particularly honored and organized in a rigid hierarchy, along with officials and priests.

      ❂   ❂   ❂

The great civilizations that flourished in what is now known politically as Iraq, and geographically as Mesopotamia, the land lying between the Euphrates and the Tigris rivers, are of about the same age as the Egyptian civilization. Ancient Mesopotamia did not have the political unity and continuity found in the Nile valley. A southern empire, Sumer, overcame the northern empire of Akkad, to be replaced after its victory by the southern empire of Babylon, which in turn was opposed by the northern empire of Assyria. But in spite of these political vagaries, there is basically one Mesopotamian civilization, which is often loosely called Babylonian.

Medical documents from this region are far more numerous than those from Egypt. The ancient Mesopotamians wrote on clay tablets that have survived far better than papyrus. On the other hand, Mesopotamian documents are far less orderly, far more casual, and much shorter than Egyptian documents. This suggests that they were mere notes which helped to maintain an extensive oral tradition. Physicians' seals, which may also have served as amulets, reveal the existence of physicians in the Sumerian Empire as early as 3000 B.C. The oldest surviving legal code, the code of King Hammurabi of Babylon (about 2250 B.C.) probably goes back to Sumerian laws which are a thousand years older. It contained, among many other legal regulations, laws specifying fees for medical practice and punishments in case of malpractice. "If the doctor shall treat a gentleman and shall open an abscess with the knife and shall preserve the eye of the patient, he shall receive ten shekels of silver. If the patient is a slave his master shall pay two shekels of silver. If the doctor shall open an abscess with a blunt knife and shall kill the patient or shall destroy the sight of the eye, his hand shall be cut off." [3] In the case of a slave, "he shall replace the slave with another slave." These legal provisions testify to the practice of surgery at an early stage. They also talk of "healers of beef and ass," that is, veterinarians.

In Mesopotamia, as in Egypt, medicine centered round religion. Numerous gods and goddesses controlled health and disease. Apparently all physicians, exorcists, diviners, and surgeons belonged to the priestly class. Even the wet nurses seem to have been recruited from the ranks of the clergy, in this case from the sacred prostitutes. Again information is most easily attainable about court physicians, who were organized in a well-ordered hierarchy.

The disease theory of the Mesopotamians was a religious one. Disease was the punishment of sin, resulting in a state of impurity or uncleanliness. All four notions—disease, sin, punishment of sin, and uncleanliness—were so close in meaning that they could sometimes be expressed by the same term. When a mortal committed a sin, which might be no more than a violation of one of the numerous food or other taboos, the gods retracted their protection from him, and he fell a prey to the innumerable disease-bearing devils and ghosts which swarmed around Mesopotamia. A sorcerer, too, could afflict his fellow men with devils.

The disease was sometimes so obviously the work of a certain devil that no further diagnosis was necessary. In more complicated cases, the priest recited a long list of possible sins to the patient in the hope that he might be able to choose from this list the sin that had produced his disease. If both methods failed, divination entered the scene.

To be obsessed with the future seems a common human trait. But hardly any other civilization appears to have suffered from this obsession to the extent that the Mesopotamians did. The number of divination methods used by the ancient Mesopotamians is almost unlimited. All of them might be applied in the diagnosis of disease. Only a few of the most important ones can be mentioned here. In a country with a highly developed astronomy, astrology of course stood in the first rank of divination methods. Hepatoscopy, that is, divining from the shape and the consistency of the liver of a sacrificial animal, induced Mesopotamian priests to construct for the instruction of novices the curious and rather accurate liver models that have been discovered by archeologists. It is significant that this detailed knowledge of the liver, acquired for supernaturalistic reasons, did not lead to any further development of anatomical knowledge among the Mesopotamians.

Dreams, which have had a recent comeback in medicine, were widely used for divination. Also used were abnormal births in man and animals, a custom which quite incidentally has provided modern research with some early data on teratology, the science of monstrosities. Equally revealing for the physician-priest was the behavior of animals, fire, rivers, plants, and oil on a watery surface.

Therapeutics were strongly colored by these religious concepts. Confession and sacrifice with prayers were necessary to appease the gods. Amulets served as prophylactics. Magic spells, sometimes highly poetic, were able to drive out the evil spirits:

> Seven are they, seven are they,
> In the Ocean Deep seven are they,
> Battening in Heaven seven are they,
> In the Ocean Deep as their home they were reared,
> Nor male or female are they,
> They are as the roaming windblast,
> No wife have they, no son do they beget;
> Knowing neither mercy nor pity,
> They hearken not unto prayer or supplication.
> They are as horses reared among the hills;
> The Evil Ones of Ea,
> Throne-bearers to the gods are they.
> They stand in the highway to befoul the path,
> Evil are they, evil are they,
> Seven are they, seven are they,
> Twice seven are they!
> By Heaven be ye exorcised! By Earth be ye exorcised![4]

Yet Mesopotamian medicine also made a start toward transcending this purely supernatural approach. A certain number of tablets are extant which contain a short description of a disease, a diagnosis, and a prescription of drugs and spells. Sometimes the transformation of omens into symptoms is clearly recognizable. Though these descriptions are not quite as developed as those from Egypt, the empirical approach is similar. The tablets mention diseases of the liver and the eye, respiratory diseases, fever, and gonorrhea, in the treatment of which a catheter was already used. They show some knowledge of night blindness, otitis media (inflammation of the middle ear), renal calculus, strokes, and scabies. The Mesopotamian tablets also reveal the existence of an extensive pharmacopoeia, including *Dreckapotheke*. The Mesopotamians knew hellebore, hyoscyamus, mandrake, and opium.

The virtue of cleanliness was practiced widely. Admirable sewage systems, and even water closets four thousand years

---

[4] Quoted in R. Campbell Thompson, *The Devils of Ancient Babylonia* (London, 1903), p. 77.

of age, have been dug out by archeologists. The notion of contagion, isolation of lepers, and regular rest days, which came into modern culture through the ancient Jews, seem to have been of Mesopotamian origin. So far, all attempts to find Egyptian or Mesopotamian origins for Greek medical practices have failed.

*   *   *

Information concerning the ancient civilizations of Central and South America is even less definitive than that on the ancient civilizations of the Old World. Yet there are good reasons for believing that, in spite of the absence of such fundamentals as domestic animals and wheeled vehicles, the level of civilization, and in particular the level of medical achievement, reached by these cultures was not inferior to the accomplishments of the Old World. Information on these civilizations must be drawn mainly from the Spanish chroniclers and their Indian pupils. The Mayan hieroglyphs and the Peruvian quipus have not been deciphered, and the Mexican Aztecs' pictographic codices can be interpreted only to a limited degree. The Spanish conquerors were full of praise for the medicine of the conquered. Cortez, for instance, wrote that European physicians were not needed in the new country. This compliment for Aztec medicine is a poor reflection on sixteenth-century European medicine. The king of Spain dispatched his own body physician, Hernandez, to Mexico in order to study the medicine of the Aztecs. Hernandez spent seven years in such studies. Unfortunately only a part of his results has been preserved.

Mexican medicine, like that of Egypt and Mesopotamia, centered round religion. The king was priest as well as political head. There were gods of disease and of healing. The concepts of sin as a cause of disease, and confession as a treatment of it, were highly developed. Astrology was used in the diagnosis of disease, and sorcery was fought with amulets and incantations. But the concept of disease-bringing winds, originally entirely religious (the wind gods bringing disease), opened the door for more rational developments. The existence of a certain empiricism is also evidenced in the numerous disease names.

Most impressive is the knowledge of and the interest in natural history in ancient Mexico. The Aztecs knew of twelve hundred medicinal plants, their knowledge being particularly rich in the field of narcotics. The Aztec king had his own botanical garden, filled primarily with medicinal plants. It is quite possible that in this field, as in the field of zoological gardens, he served as a model for European sovereigns. Such extensive knowledge of natural history is conducive to the beginnings of classification. On the other hand, it is remarkable that there is no evidence of any high grade of anatomical knowledge in ancient Mexico, in spite of the fact that human sacrifice offered rich opportunities for observing human anatomy. Surgery seems to have been better developed than in most primitive societies. The Mexicans practiced suture with hair, embryotomy, and other operations. Fumigation, baths, bloodletting, diet, and other physical methods were widely used.

There is evidence of a great deal of specialization in Mexican medicine. In addition to general practitioners, there were diviners, surgeons, phlebotomists, pharmacists, and physicians specializing in various diseases. At least some of the specialties were open to women practitioners. In general the specialization appears to have stemmed from a survival of primitive practices rather than from technical advances. The Mexican hospitals represented an important advance in the field of medical care.

*   *   *

The ancient Peruvian civilization, of which the Inca Empire was only a relatively recent offshoot, offers many parallels with Mexico and the ancient cultures of the Near East. The fragmentary nature of the information supplied by chroniclers is particularly obvious in the case of Peru. Here surgery was obviously very highly developed; yet no written record exists to verify the performance of such extensive operations as trephining and amputations. Gods and sorcerers were regarded as disease-causing agents, and confessions and exorcisms were thought of as appropriate countermeasures. The magic rite of transference of disease to animals, known in many primitive societies, seems to have been particularly widespread in Peru. This transference was practiced mainly upon the guinea pig, which seems thus to have started its painful career in medicine. The concept of disease-bringing winds was developed into an insight into the seasonal occurrence of disease. This insight represents a first step toward the recognition of natural law. The ancient Peruvians not only domesticated one of the most important crops on earth, the potato, but also contributed such valuable substances as cocaine and Peruvian balm to our pharmacopeia.

The most spectacular accomplishments of the ancient Peruvians undoubtedly lay in the field of surgery. The Peruvians were able to carry out such difficult operations as trepanation, amputation, and the excision of tumors. Even prostheses were known. As in other parts of South America and in the Old World, the heads of ants were used as clamps in sutures. Our information on Peruvian surgery stems chiefly from their pottery. Peruvian pottery of the Chimu period deserves to be counted among the greatest works of art of all times. It is fortunate for medical historians that Peruvian artists exhibited a somewhat morbid inclination to represent disease in their pottery. This pottery shows surgical operations and the consequences of ritual and judiciary mutilations. It gives a clear picture of the ravages following *uta*, the leishmaniasis resulting from infection by local parasitic organisms. It also depicts the dangerous local Rickettsia disease, called verruga peruana or Carrión's disease. For a while it was hotly debated whether some of the vessels portrayed cases of syphilis or leprosy. Most students of the problem have now settled on leishmaniasis.

It was natural that the totalitarian Inca state, which left nothing to accident, should have had to its credit special accomplishments in the field of public health. An annual health ceremony, *Citua*, under the leadership of the Inca, provided an occasion for a thorough cleaning of all homes. Provision was made for the appropriate upkeep and employment of the aged and crippled, and marriage of the latter was restricted. Alcoholism and drug addiction were energetically fought.

Like modern totalitarians, the ancient Incas practiced the transfer of populations on a large scale. But the Incas showed considerable hygienic insight in their population transfers. They realized that those of their subjects who had grown up under extreme highland conditions would not survive settlement in the tropical lowlands. Accordingly, populations were transferred only to locations corresponding climatically to their former settlements. In the same way, highland troops were never kept more than a few months in lowland conditions. The impressive ruins of bathing establishments and sewage systems testify to the ability of the Incas in public health engineering.

One of the most remarkable actions of the Incas in the field of medicine was their attempt to overcome primitive specialization. It was particularly the Inca Pachacutec who demanded that future physicians as well as surgeons should have a solid background in herbalism.

        ✿   ✿   ✿

In the above treatment of medicine of four ancient civilizations, all four systems of medicine are regarded as expressions of a certain general type of medicine, that which has been called "archaic medicine" by Temkin. But does such a type really exist? Is it not too easy to be carried away by enthusiasm for these civilizations and to invest their medicine, so closely akin to primitive medicine, with special virtues which do not really exist?

There seems little doubt that these medical systems do not contain any single trait that is not also contained to some degree in the medicine of primitives. The complete independence of medicine from supernaturalism was not achieved in any of them. Practitioners remained priests, and supernaturalism remained the dominant element in medicine. Nevertheless, on the basis of the evidence presented it seems safe to state that the high degree of empiricism, scientific systematization, and practical organization—shown, for instance, in the overcoming of primitive specialization—make it reasonable to talk of a new and different type of medicine.

It is true that this new type exhibits far more quantitative than qualitative differences. It is primarily the result of general developments, not of special medical discoveries. The mere fact that medical experiences were now written down, collected, and transmitted by priestly organizations made possible a tremendous increase in the field of experience and a rapid diffusion of techniques and technical ability. Every single operation performed by Peruvian surgeons also has been practiced by at least one primitive tribe. But, while the primitives knew just one or two particular operations, the Peruvians developed a real surgery through the combination of the different surgical abilities and skills over a large area. Again, the congregation of large populations almost inevitably results in public health measures. While small primitive communities may survive without such measures, every large concentration of population would be wiped out by disease if it did not develop some technique of public health. The emphasis on public health is another distinguishing feature of this newer type of medicine.

Chapter 4

ANCIENT INDIA AND CHINA

Although the ancient civilizations have died out, the Oriental civilizations of the river valleys of India and China have survived up to the present time. And their systems of medicine have survived with them. Thousands of practitioners still apply these ancient types of medicine to millions of patients. A knowledge of these medical systems and their history is thus of immediate practical importance, for successful introduction of modern scientific medicine into these countries depends on sympathetic and tactful handling of the old. In both countries medicine developed beyond the stage of archaic priest medicine before eventually becoming static. In both countries the medical profession became truly independent. This change in status was, significantly enough, paid for by a lowering of the social rank of the medical practitioner. In neither country did medicine reach the stage of modern scientific medicine. It often showed in its subservience to a rather dogmatic philosophy a striking similarity to the medieval medicine of Western civilizations.

❀ ❀ ❀

The history of Indian medicine is divided into two great periods. An earlier one, lasting until about 800 B.C., is called the Vedic period, because information concerning the medicine of this period is derived mainly from the Vedas, the four holy Sanskrit books of the Indians. A later period, the Brahmanic, roughly covers the period from 800 B.C. to A.D. 1000, after which time large parts of India were submitted to Islamic rule and Arab doctors took over medical practice in many places. This second period in Indian medicine is called Brahmanic because it was based on a culture ideologically dominated by the Brahmanic caste, the caste of Hindu priests.

What little is known of the medicine of the Vedic period shows that it closely resembled primitive and archaic medicine. The familiar concepts stand out—sin as the cause of disease, confession as a healing rite, and demons to be fought by exorcisms, spells, and hymns. The existence of a great many diseases is reflected in the Vedic books. As might be expected, fevers predominate, for India is still probably the most malarial country on earth as well as a breeding ground for plague and cholera. Even in this early period the Hindus showed a marked predilection for purifying treatments with water. Their unusual skill in surgery is made evident by their use of prostheses.

Doctors in the Brahmanic period belonged to a third caste, lower in rank than the priest and the warrior castes. They used helpers from still lower castes. The doctor's education did not take place in priest schools, but through apprenticeship. The approach was primarily rational, and medical education was of a high caliber. A great deal of thought was given to proper education, proper balance of theory and practice in teaching, and proper balance between medical and surgical knowledge. The future doctor had to practice on a large number of teaching models. Introduction into the profession was marked by a solemn ceremony in which an oath, resembling the Hippocratic oath, was taken. This is only one of the many parallels between Hindu and Greek medicine. The three great classics of Brahmanic medicine are the books of Charaka (written at the beginning of the Christian Era), Susruta (about A.D. 500), and Vagbhata (about A.D. 600). These books are probably based on much older, sometimes Vedic, material. To the extent that Indian material can be dated, it seems likely that the ideas of classic Indian medicine developed between 700 and 200 B.C.

The supernatural elements in Brahmanic medicine are

still considerable. Besides humoral pathology, possession by demons or pathology through migration of the soul (Karma) are recognized. In the last case, disease is punishment for a sin committed in a former existence. The medical treatises are of divine and mythological origin. They are partly written in verse and are full of prayers. Omina are still important for prognoses.

The great religious movement of the sixth century B.C., based on the teachings of Buddha, had a powerful influence on medicine. It brought about the founding of hospitals in India many centuries before Christianity produced the same effect in the West. The close connection between religion and medicine is reflected in the fact that the traditional four questions the Indian healer asks the patient correspond largely to the "four noble truths" of Buddha.

Halfway between the scientific and the religious elements of this medicine we find the semiscientific, exemplified by astrology. The position of the patient in space, the astrological implications of a certain day, winds, and the six seasons (abnormal seasons are the consequence of sin!) play an important role in Indian medical thought.

This thought is, like Greek or Chinese, based above all on an extensive speculative science. This science recognises the existence of five basic principles (earth, water, fire, air, sky), two qualities (hot and cold), three humors (air, bile, and phlegm), six body elements (chyle, blood, flesh, bone, marrow, semen), and the so-called vital force.

According to this theory all diseases are originally humoral disturbances. Symptoms are caused by too little or too much of the body humors and body elements. The same change does not always cause the same symptom. Psychosomatic considerations occur frequently. Dissections are recommended, but anatomical knowledge is poor.

A subdivision of medicine as found in Susruta strikes us as strange, but in many ways it is quite significant. It goes as follows: (1) removal of foreign bodies, (2) diseases above the clavicle, (3) general diseases (fever, hysteria, leprosy, and so on), (4) diseases caused by demons, (5) pediatrics, (6) toxicology, (7) rejuvenation, (8) aphrodisiaca. We should not forget that our Christian-Hebrew attitude towards sexuality was unknown and incomprehensible to Asiatics as well as to the ancient Greeks.

The following disease causes are mentioned in the classic Indian books: faulty semen or ovum and wrong behavior of the mother during pregnancy, producing deaf, blind, and idiotic children; so-called idiopathic diseases of body or mind; traumatism; seasonal diseases; diseases caused by demons or gods; "spontaneous diseases" (diseases caused by old age, hunger, thirst, and so on).

Diagnostics were highly developed. The Indian healer used questioning, very thorough inspection (e.g., to diagnose pulmonary consumption from loss of weight), touch (including observation of the pulse), and examination with other senses, such as tasting the urine for diabetes. Indians knew the sweet taste of diabetic urine long before Europeans did. In diagnostics, many different kinds of pain were taken into consideration.

Brahmanic physicians believed strongly in the role of constitution, of body build; they believed they knew the external signs of longevity. They observed the proportions of the body and differentiated seven temperaments. Age was another important element of their calculations, as were the seasons. They divided India into three climatic regions.

Like the Hippocratic school they were prognosis-minded. Omina had been replaced by prognostic signs. They, too, knew the Hippocratic plucking of the covering by the dying. They regarded changes in sense perception and the "retreat of the penis into the body" as very important. (Still, under the name of "Koro," an important disease in Java. This occurs, strangely enough, in Auenbrugger). They knew that the prognosis of ulcera in leprosy, tuberculosis, and diabetes was poor.

Prognosis was very important, since Indian healers in general did not treat incurables. Their books abound in warnings against such action.

The clinical knowledge of the classic Indian physician was very extensive. He knew bloodspitting in pulmonary consumption. Leprosy was regarded as contagious. He knew the carbuncles of diabetics and the ascites of liver disease.

Fevers were, of course, one of the main concerns. They knew the different forms of malaria, and some Buddhist writings betray an awareness of the role of mosquitoes. The ancient Indians also knew about the fact that plague epidemics are preceded by rats dying in great quantities. Their books contain excellent descriptions of epilepsy and other convulsive disorders, of tetanus, hemiplegia, elephantiasis, and erysipelas. Under the heading "abscesses," they also discuss puerperal fever and osteomyelitis, and they try to differentiate abscesses from tumors. They separate goiter and scrofulosis. Alcoholism and mental diseases are treated physically as well as psychologically. General diseases are dealt with extensively.

The ancient Indian physicians were apparently almost obsessed with classifications. Susruta, e.g., enumerates 66 diseases of the oral cavity and 5 of the earlobe. Thus, a very luxuriant nomenclature grew up, even without the benefit of Latin or Greek.

All forms of therapeutics, including surgery, are accompanied by prayers or spells. Against bad dreams temple sleep is prescribed. The center of therapeutics is diet. Food and its properties are examined very closely. Certain foods are incompatible. In hydropsy a salt-free diet is indicated. Numerous emetics, cathartics, venesection, and leeches cleanse the patient's body and soul. The abuse of cathartics and emetics can produce no less than 15 diseases.

In spite of emphasizing diet, ancient Indian medicine developed a very extensive pharmacopoeia. Certain soils were regarded as particularly suitable for certain herbs. Herbs can be classified according to their qualities or their taste, according to the five elements, or according to their effect. The drugs are either of mineral, animal, or plant origin. The main liquid drugs are water, milk, wine, or the urine of the elephant cow. The prescriptions are composed of many elements (polypharmacy) and are often accompanied by quackish claims of absolute efficacy, such as for iron against leprosy or as a diabetes panacea. The substances can be applied orally or as poultices, fumigations, snuff, or gargling solutions or can be introduced into rectum, bladder, or vagina. The fame of Indian drugs was always great, and they were adopted by the Egyptians, Greeks, Arabs, and western Europeans. The last named also showed a tremendous appetite for Indian spices, which brought about during the fifteenth century the discovery of the maritime routes from western Europe to India via South Africa. Quite recently, the elements of an Indian herb, Rauwolfia serpentina, have been incorporated with great success into our own pharmacopoeia.

The Indians knew many poisons from the mineral, plant, and animal kingdoms. They suffered much from snakebite, poisoned missiles, and insect and rat bites. They had developed certain chemical skills, and differentiated acids and alkalis.

Even more remarkable is the spirit in which drugs were applied. In Susruta we read the important statement that the remedy should not be stronger than the patient or the disease. He knows four elements of a treatment: the physician, the patient, the remedy, and the nurse. It is typical that he is energetically opposed to innovations, to the search for new drugs. Tradition suffices.

The most brilliant achievement of the Indians was undoubtedly their surgery, the so-called "removal of foreign bodies." Each operation was initiated by a prayer. The patient was laid in the "right" direction, and astrology was consulted. Then one of the following eight techniques was applied: incision, excision, scraping, puncturing, probing, extraction, provoking secretion, or suturing. The high standards of Indian surgery are reflected in the fact that the sequelae of faulty operations are extensively and honestly discussed. One hundred different instruments were available, but the hand was regarded as the most important. The surgeon had to know the art of exhilarating as well as intimidating the patient. Among the instruments, tongs, rectal specula, bougies, hooks for nasal polyps, and the magnet are mentioned. Cauterization with the hot iron and chemosurgery with caustic salves were practiced. A great number of bandages and bandaging materials were known. When it was a matter of cupping, horns were used for wind, leeches for bile, and gourds for phlegm. Venesection and scarification were applied. Wine served as an anesthetic. Around 1840, the British surgeon James Esdaile (1808–1859) brought back from India hypnosis as an anesthetic technique. It did not take root, since the chemical anesthetics were discovered simultaneously in the United States.

It is no accident that Susruta's catalog of operations begins with piercing the earlobes, a typical magical procedure. The acme of Indian surgery is undoubtedly reached in the plastic operations of ear and nose. Frequent punitive mutilations of these organs offered many opportunities for the surgeon to develop his technique. There is little doubt that plastic surgery in Europe, which flourished first in medieval Italy, is a direct descendant of classic Indian surgery. Remarkable also were Indian accomplishments in the fields of cataract and stone operations, and the suturing of the intestine with the heads of large ants as clamps. During the numberless wars a fine technique of missile extraction was developed. Fifteen different modalities were known including the use of the magnet. Those spots of the body that are of vital importance were specially studied.

Of burns four degrees were differentiated. Treatment of wounds, fractures, and luxations was very competent. Indian surgeons operated for tumors, mastitis, scrofulosis, goiter, hydrocele, and hernias. Special attention was given to operating on hemorrhoids, polyps, anal fistulas, the stone, and intestinal occlusion. There was in existence a highly developed treatment of diseases of eyes, ears, and nose.

Indian obstetrics were a queer mixture of instructions on

how to make a male child, of pseudoembryology, signs of pregnancy, diets in pregnancy, and discussions of some false presentations and some maneuvers.

The ancient Indians put great emphasis on hygiene and prevention. They recommended toothbrushing, chewing of betel leaves, anointing, combing, exercise, massage, bathing, piety, taking the proper food, sitting idle, sexual intercourse (once in four days), politeness, not being witness or guarantor, not going to crossroads, not urinating in the presence of superiors, cows, or against the wind, not sleeping during the daytime, and not eating fly-infested food. During epidemics one should not drink water or eat raw vegetables; one should run away and pray. Lest we smile at this strange mixture of Indian hygienic measures, we might remember that the Indians knew for thousands of years a technique for preventing smallpox, which the Europeans learned from the Turks only during the eighteenth century: inoculation.

The total configuration of Indian classic medicine suggests some comparisons and parallels. Indian medicine reminds us of archaic medicine, but it is more scientific. Indian medicine enormously resembles Greek medicine in regard to its scientific principles as well as its technology. The Indians were often even better technicians. On the other hand, the Greeks achieved a complete separation of medicine and religion, never obtained by the Indians, and the Greeks never pressed their medicine into one rigid, systematic framework.

Indian medicine also has much in common with medieval medicine. We observe here the same mixing of religion and systematized science, but the Indians were far better empiricists and were extremely successful just in the field of surgery, which reached its lowest ebb in our own Middle Ages.

It is very unlikely that the Indians learned their medicine from the Greeks of Alexander the Great during the fourth century B.C. By this time, it seems, Indian medicine was already well advanced. It had developed partly independently of, partly before, Greek medicine, but it had never separated from religion. The Greeks probably received many suggestions from India via Persia, and the Indians probably received Greek stimuli the same way. It was a Greek characteristic to pick up cultural elements everywhere and to develop them then in a dynamic way instead of remaining static.

When Europe became static and religious during the Middle Ages, its medicine resembled Indian medicine tremendously, except that Indian medicine was much better. When in Europe, through the Renaissance, the Greek attitude prevailed again, Europe surpassed India rapidly. The Arabs, the Greeks, and other Europeans were not the only ones to learn from India. Indian culture and therewith Indian medicine spread just as much in an eastern direction, as is evident from Tibetan, Indochinese, and Indonesian medicine.

      *   *   *

China is undoubtedly the youngest of the old civilizations, although recent archeological findings of early Chinese "bone cultures" make the traditional Chinese historical data appear more plausible than they seemed a few decades ago. Despite its apparently static character, Chinese civilization has shown a great deal of technological inventiveness. The Chinese apparently knew of the compass as early as 1100 B.C. They used silk, porcelain, and printing long before these were known in the West. Theirs was an extremely literate society, where even the gods were addressed by letter, and scholars ran the administration. The doctor, unfortunately, did not belong to the scholastic group, at least in the later periods of Chinese history, and did not share in the general respect paid to the scholar.

Chinese medical literature is very extensive. The beginnings of medicine are credited to three legendary emperors: Fu-Hsi (according to Chinese tradition about 2900 B.C.), who invented the fundamental philosophy of *yang* and *yin*,

the male and the female principles in nature; Shen-Nung
(about 2700 B.C.), who invented drug lore and acupuncture;
and Huang-ti (about 2600 B.C.), who is supposed to be the
author of *Neiching*, the classic book on internal diseases.

Anatomy and physiology are largely of a fanciful and de-
ductive character. Medicine is entirely dominated by an
extremely formalized and elaborate natural philosophy.
Simultaneously, especially for the lower strata of the population, there exists a kind of supernaturalistic priest medicine, or shamanism, based on the primitive theory of soul
abduction.

According to Chinese philosophy and science, the whole
universe is divided into two principles, *yang* (light, male),
and *yin* (dark, female). There are five basic elements (wood,
fire, earth, metal, water) associated with five planets, five di-
rections, five seasons, five colors, five sounds, and five organs
in the human body. Characteristically enough, music is
thought of as the science of sciences. Disease is regarded as
a disharmony between the five fundamental organs, a disharmony which is in turn connected with the interference of
the planets, seasons, colors, and sounds corresponding with
each organ.

Diagnosis is based primarily on observation of the pulse
and inspection of the tongue. There are no less than fifty-one
different types of pulse, and thirty-seven different shades of
the tongue are described. A great deal of sound clinical observation is incorporated into this system of medicine. For
instance, the itch mite is known, and diabetes, smallpox,
dysentery, measles, and cholera are well described. Yet the
system as a whole, like that of India, is impaired by over-
elaboration. To take only one example, the Chinese doctor
has to distinguish between no less than forty-two forms of
smallpox. The Chinese, too, knew the prevention of this disease through inoculation. They were also aware of the connection between a high rat mortality and plague epidemics.

The pharmacopeia is very highly developed. It contains
as many as eighteen hundred drugs, and in recent times such

valuable remedies as ephedrine, chaulmoogra oil, and buffa-gin have been taken over from the Chinese by Western medicine. At a much earlier date rhubarb and camphor probably came into the European pharmacopeia from the Chinese. The Chinese also use cod-liver oil and mineral sub-stances such as iron, arsenic, and mercury. The doctor's pre-scriptions are filled in regular drugstores, and among the "dragon bones"—the bones of prehistoric animals sold in Chinese drug stores—some of the most important fossils dis-covered in recent years have been found by von Koenigswald.

Because of a deeply rooted aversion in their culture to the shedding of blood, combined with a belief that mutilation continues in the life after death, surgery has never developed among the Chinese, in spite of their considerable knowledge of anesthetics and their otherwise extensive adoption of Hindu medical practices. However, physiotherapy is very highly developed. In addition to methods known everywhere —such as dry cupping, massage, and gymnastics—the Chinese invented two methods of their own, namely, acupuncture and moxa. The technique of acupuncture with long needles is based on the idea that the body is full of canal-like tubes, which have to be made permeable again. This is a natural idea to the Chinese since their agriculture was based on irri-gation. Acupuncture has appeared periodically in Western medicine during the last three centuries. Like many other fads, it probably works through suggestion. Moxa, in which the patient is burned with cones of dried herbs, has not appealed to European practitioners or patients.

It is characteristic of Chinese civilization that a well-or-ganized legal medicine existed as early as in the thirteenth century A.D. While many of the tests employed were rather fantastic, fingerprints were used for identification of crimi-nals. Public health was not well developed, and the dirt of Chinese cities is proverbial. The original thirteen specialties of earlier times were reduced in the course of time to nine. The practice of smallpox inoculation was probably imported from India. Both medicines, the Indian and Chinese, froze relatively early into rigid dogmatism and continued in this static form throughout the centuries to the present time. Because of the impossibility of providing a population of over a billion with scientifically trained physicians, the Communist Chinese government now uses traditional practitioners and so-called barefoot doctors, who receive three months' training. These are also responsible for disease prevention.

It is interesting that the Japanese, who took over Chinese medicine together with Chinese culture in the ninth century A.D., did not show the same conservatism. During the sixteenth century, probably under the stimulus of foreign contact, they developed a more direct clinical approach and a greater reliance on the healing forces of nature. Nagata Tokuhon, known as the Japanese Hippocrates, played an important part in these developments. Under Western influence the Japanese made great progress in surgery in the seventeenth century, and in obstetrics and anatomy in the eighteenth. In the second half of the nineteenth century they were able to assimilate Western medicine as a whole with great ease and skill (see Chap. 15).

Chapter 5

GREEK MEDICINE: PHYSICIANS, PRIESTS, PHILOSOPHERS

Ancient Greek medicine is incomparably closer to modern medicine than any other historical form of medicine. This is hardly surprising, since modern medicine would not exist without the Greek precedent. It is no accident that modern medical terminology is to such a large extent based on Greek. There are, of course, numerous differences between present-day medicine and Greek medicine, even as there are variations within Greek medicine itself. It must be remembered that Greek medicine covered a period of about one thousand years, and that, far from being static, it was in a ferment of continuous change and ebullition. Yet the successive epochs of Greek medicine have one thing in common with each other and with the medicine of modern times. Disease was no longer regarded as a supernatural phenomenon; it was approached from a rational, naturalistic, and scientific point of view.

It has never been fully explained why all of a sudden, more than twenty-five hundred years ago, a small group of people in the Eastern Mediterranean took this important and radical step in human thought. But several contributing factors can be named. Because of their geographical location, the Greeks were exposed to the most varied cultural contacts. They came under the influence of the Egyptian, Mesopotamian, Phoenician, and Cretan civilizations. All these civilizations contained certain elements which could contribute to the new approach, and their very multiplicity, with the contradictions involved, may have provoked a new departure.

Intellectually and physically the Greeks showed what genet-
icists call "hybrid vigor." The extreme political division
which prevailed in Greece throughout her history, and which
was eventually to be her undoing, prevented the development of the strong and well-organized priest bureaucracy
which had maintained its hold on thought and practice in
other civilizations. Individualism and critical thought could
develop, at least in the upper classes, to a degree unattain-
able in the Oriental empires.

Not that religious medicine was unknown to the Greeks.
It was very prominent in earlier times, and for many, especially the poor and the incurables, medicine retained its religious orientation throughout Greek history. The Greek
physicians who treated the upper class were themselves no
disbelievers, but were naturalists who separated their practice from their religious beliefs.

The Greeks had many gods, and many of these gods took
a hand in producing and curing disease. In the course of time
Apollo was regarded more and more as the god of disease
and healing, until in the fifth century B.C. he was replaced by
Asclepius, whose staff and holy snake are still the symbols
of the medical profession. Asclepius had his temples all over
the ancient world, first in Greece and Asia Minor, and later
in Rome and the Roman possessions. In his temples the patient was treated by "incubation"; he slept a night in the
temple of the god, and during his sleep the god would appear
to him and prescribe for him. The inscriptions from these
temples give abundant documentation for this form of
healing. A typical votive inscription reads as follows:

Erasippe from Kaphy: She slept in the temple and dreamt that the
God applied massage to her stomach and kissed her and gave her a
cup containing a drug. He commanded her to drink it and then to
vomit. She did so and soiled her garment. When she woke up in the
morning, she saw her garment full of the filth she had vomited, and
thereupon she recovered.

There was, thus, an extensive segment of Greek medicine
that was closely connected with religion. But it is now gen-

erally agreed that Asclepius, originally a legendary physician and a patron of the guild of physicians, became a god
only during the fifth century B.C., between 475 and 425. Thus
the outstanding type of Greek temple medicine was not the
predecessor but the contemporary of classic Greek medicine.
Hippocrates supposedly lived from 460 to 377 B.C., and the
treatises of the Hippocratic collection, the *Corpus Hippocraticum*, are supposed to have been written between 480 and
380 B.C. It can therefore no longer be maintained that the
Hippocratic physicians were the successors and pupils of the
priests of Asclepius, nor that the temple inscriptions are the
first "case histories." By the time Asclepius rose to the rank
of a god and his cult had become widespread, the independent physicians and philosopher-scientists were already firmly
established. The title of Asclepiad, which some of the physicians used, has produced much confusion. But it is now clear
that this title did not refer to the god or to a religious corpora-
tion, but to certain guilds or families of physicians.

Independent physicians appear in the writings of Homer
(about 1000 B.C.), and no mention of priest-physicians is made
there. The physicians in Homer are all independent and respected craftsmen. Asclepius himself, and his sons Machaon
and Podalirius, are chieftains who, like many other chieftains,
are skilled in treating wounds. Medicine in Homer consists
almost entirely of military surgery, since his epics deal mostly
with warfare.

It seems that by the seventh century a medical tradition
had developed in Cnidus, a Greek settlement in Asia Minor.
The names of Euryphon and Ctesias have been transmitted
to us as outstanding representatives of this school. The school
of Cnidus was apparently concerned primarily with the diagnosis of disease, developing a somewhat elaborate system of
classification. Cnidian physicians differentiated no less than
twelve forms of cystitis. The treatment of these Cnidians
was active and primarily local. Apparently, they resorted
more easily to surgical interventions than did the Coans.
The school which grew up on the island of Cos during the
sixth century, and which has been immortalized through the

name of Hippocrates and the books of the Hippocratic collection, was, on the contrary, primarily interested in prognosis and in general treatment. A third medical group developed in Crotona, Sicily, during the fifth century, and there were apparently flourishing schools in Rhodes and Cyrene. It is noteworthy that all these early centers grew up, not on the Greek mainland, but in the colonies on the periphery of Greek civilization. This supports the theory that foreign stimuli played a great role in the development of Greek thought. The "schools" here mentioned were groups held together by the same tradition, not active teaching institutions. The Greek physician was a craftsman and therefore was trained not in school but through apprenticeship to an individual master. Among craftsmen he was the most respected since he dealt with health, and the Greek interest in health was almost hypochondriac. If he was not salaried by a city administration, he had to migrate from one city to another. The upper crust on which he lived was in general too thin to keep him alive permanently in one given locality.

The life of Democedes, a physician of the sixth century, illustrates the peripatetic existence of the Greek physician. Born and raised in Crotona, Democedes went to Aegina as a city physician. Then he accepted a more rewarding position in Athens. He left Athens to become the body physician of the tyrant Polycrates of Samos. There he was captured by the Persian emperor Darius, who also used him as a body physician. Through an ingenious scheme he succeeded in escaping from Persia and returned to his home town of Crotona, which toward the end of his life he had to leave again because of political difficulties.

The great interest of the Greeks in athletics led to the creation of gymnasiums. The "coaches" in these gymnasiums, the gymnasts, had a good opportunity to develop medical knowledge through their experience with accidents. They also advanced medical techniques in the field of physiotherapy.

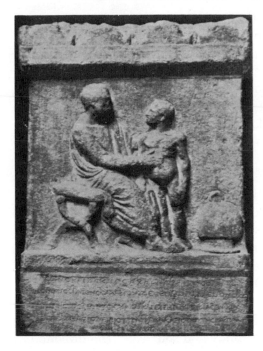

FIGURE 3. Greek physician palpating.

Of decisive importance for the development of Greek medicine was the mutual influence of philosophy and medicine. Greek natural philosophy provides one of the great landmarks in the evolution of human thought. For man to think systematically at all was undoubtedly a great step forward. But strangely enough his first systematized thoughts had not centered around earthly things, but around spirits and gods. Now, in the seventh century B.C., for the first time man emancipated himself from supernaturalistic thought and tried to understand the world on a natural basis. Of course, such thought was necessarily incomplete and speculative. Nevertheless it contained astonishing insights, some of which are still basic to human thinking. Crude as the first theories were, they brought order to an infinite diversity of phenomena. Any feelings of superiority toward these speculations should be tempered by the realization that even today basic scientific assumptions such as the theory of evolution are still of a hypothetical nature. An important aspect of these early speculations was the fact that they were continually submitted to criticism rather than being frozen into religious dogmas. It is remarkable that early Greek philosophy, like early medicine, originated on the periphery of Greek civilization. This fact once again points up the role played by outside stimuli in the formation of Greek thought.

Only a few fragments survive concerning the ideas of the early Greek philosophers. These give the impression that the primary goal of these speculative scientists was to find one basic element which would explain the functioning of the material world. Thales of Miletus (639–544 B.C.), who predicted the solar eclipse of May 28, 585 B.C., regarded moisture as the fundamental element; Anaximenes of Miletus (570–500 B.C.) claimed this role for air; and Heraclitus of Ephesus (556–460 B.C.) chose fire. Pythagoras of Samos (580–489 B.C.), a many-sided genius who is remembered for his mathematical work and his discovery of the first acoustic laws, transcended philosophy and science in the direction of mysticism and religion. This aspect of his thinking reflected an Egyptian influence. His emphasis on the symbolical importance of numbers is perhaps partially responsible for the elaborate lore of "critical days" in Greek medicine. This idea of "critical days" implies that diseases enter a decisive stage on either the fourth, seventh, eleventh, fourteenth, or seventeenth day. Pythagoras taught at Crotona in southern Italy, at the western end of the Greek world, and he probably had a strong influence on the Sicilian medical schools.

Empedocles of Agrigentum (504–433 B.C.) also worked in Sicily. He was probably the originator of the theory that replaced the one fundamental element of the former philosophers with four: air, fire, water, and earth. Empedocles imagined that the elements came into being through a combination of the four fundamental qualities: hot, dry, wet, and cold (see accompanying diagram). A further step was to identify the four basic elements with the four constituent humors of the body: blood, phlegm, yellow bile, and black

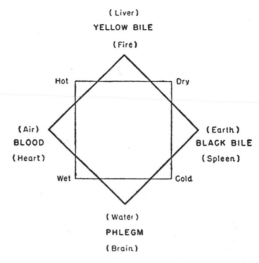

Diagram illustrating the Greek theory of the four qualities, the four elements, and the four humors. The elements were regarded as being related to qualities, and these in turn governed the respective humors. Imbalance in the qualities and humors could be compensated by using drugs associated with the opposite qualities.

bile. These four humors originated in the heart, brain, liver, and spleen respectively. This theory, through its incorporation into Hippocratic writings and its development through Aristotle and Galen, became the ruling medical theory of the Middle Ages and the following centuries. It provided the "reasons" for techniques of evacuation used long before, such as venesection, cupping, cathartics, emetics, sneezing, sweating, urination, and so on. Its popularity can probably be attributed to its simplicity. A disease of the black bile, for instance, which was "dry" and "cold," would logically be treated by "hot" and "wet" remedies.

The idea that man and the universe are composed of the same elements justifies the concept of the human body as a microcosm, which mirrors the macrocosm. The microcosm-macrocosm theory fills the history of Occidental philosophy, from the predecessors of Socrates to Paracelsus, Leibniz, and the Romantics. It became the source of numerous, mostly dubious, analogies.

During the fifth century the interest of the Greek philosophers shifted from natural toward moral philosophy. One of
the last natural philosophers, Alcmaeon of Crotona (about
500 B.C.), is one of the first Greeks known to have written on
medicine. Alcmaeon advanced the theory that disease is a
state of disequilibrium among the qualities of the body com-
ponents. At the same time, Alcmaeon was greatly interested
in anatomy and embryology. He described the optical nerve,
two kinds of blood vessels, and the trachea. He designated
the brain as the central organ of the higher activities of man.
Many ancient and later writers regarded it only as a gland
secreting phlegm. Another fifth-century philosopher, Democ-
ritus of Abdera (about 460 B.C.), deserves mention for his
theory of the atoms as minute bodies representing the ultimate unit in the physical world. Not only has this theory
been incorporated into modern science, but it also exerted
great influence on many ancient medical writers.

Chapter 6

GREEK MEDICINE: HIPPOCRATIC MEDICINE

Greek medicine was greatly influenced by the philosophers. Yet its main development was due, not to speculation, but to its practical efforts in the field of clinical observation.

The name of Hippocrates—the "father of medicine"—is a symbol of the first creative period of Greek medicine, and to a certain extent his name has come to represent the beauty, value, and dignity of medicine of all times. Paradoxically, very little is known about the life and ideas of Hippocrates of Cos (460–379 B.C.). He seems to have been the scion of a family of "Asclepiads." He traveled widely in a Greece which excelled in many fields—the philosophy of Socrates, the statesmanship of Pericles, the historical writings of Thucydides, the tragedy of Sophocles, and the sculpture of Praxiteles. Hippocrates flourished in the resplendent period between the victory of Salamis (480 B.C.), which saved Greece from the danger of Persian invasion, and the beginning of the Peloponnesian War (431 B.C.), in which the self-destruction of Greece began.

From fifty to seventy books were later attributed to Hippocrates, and in the third century B.C. they were collected in Alexandria into the *Corpus Hippocraticum*. It is not known which of these books, if any, were actually written by the great physician. As a matter of fact, none of them contains the ideas attributed to him in the writings of Plato and Menon. Some of the books are textbooks, some are monographs, and some are no more than notes; and contradictory opinions are often found in them. Thus it is clear that they are not the work of one man, or even one group. They seem to have been written between 480 and 380 B.C. While most of them express the opinions of the school of Cos, some reflect Cnidian and Sicilian teachings as well. It seems that when these works of unknown authors were eventually gathered together in Alexandria the name of Hippocrates was affixed to them, since by then Hippocrates was regarded as the greatest of the ancient physicians. Something very similar happened as late as the seventeenth century with the so-called works of Barbeyrac of Montpellier. In spite of their divergencies, the majority of the Hippocratic books have enough in common to justify speaking of "the Hippocratic physician" and "Hippocratic medicine" as definite medical types.

The *Corpus Hippocraticum* is worthy of lengthy investigation, but there is space here for a characterization of only a few of the most important books. *On Ancient Medicine* is typical of Hippocratic writings in deriving the whole art of medicine from dietetic observations and practices. The author of this book was apparently an old-fashioned empiricist and craftsman who was attacking the use of the new-fangled theory of the four qualities brought into medicine from philosophy. Consistent with this high regard for diet, the *Corpus Hippocraticum* contains several other books dealing exclusively with this subject. Diet is often understood in the larger sense as the regulation of the whole existence, not just of food intake. The famous *Epidemic Diseases*, concerned mainly with diseases of the island of Thasos, and the admirable *On Prognosis* reveal the intimate knowledge of symptoms possessed by the Hippocratic physician and give highly sophisticated descriptive detail. *On Airs, Waters, and Places* advises the physician of the diseases he will have to cope with on entering a city with given climatic conditions. In a second part of the work various countries of Europe and Asia and their institutions are interpreted in terms of climate. This book has been hailed as the first classic of medical geography, or anthropology, and it must be said that its "climatism" is far more reasonable than the "climatism" of the succeeding two thousand years in that the earlier author realizes that the effect of climatic conditions may be changed by social institution.

The surgical books, dealing with fractures, dislocations, wounds of the head, ulcers, fistulae, and hemorrhoids, are still regarded as excellent in their descriptions, though they emphasize the conservative more than the operative aspects of surgery. Majno recently noted that the books described the tourniquet. *On the Sacred Disease* makes a strong plea for the natural explanation of disease as opposed to the supernaturalistic. To the author the frightening "sacred disease" (epilepsy) is no more sacred than any other disease. The book also stresses the importance of the brain as compared with other organs such as the diaphragm. *On the Nature of Man,* an anatomical and physiological treatise, goes furthest among the Hippocratic writings in the acceptance of the theory of the four humors. The famous *Oath*[1] (according to

---

[1] I swear by Apollo the physician, and Aesculapius, and Hygieia, and Panacea, and all the gods and goddesses, that, according to my ability and judgment, I will keep this Oath and this stipulation—to reckon him who taught me this Art equally dear to me as my parents, to share my substance with him, and relieve his necessities if required; to look upon his offspring in the same footing as my own brothers, and to teach them this art, if they shall wish to learn it, without fee or stipulation; and that by precept, lecture, and every other mode of instruction, I will impart a knowledge of the Art to my own sons, and those of my teachers, and to disciples bound by a stipulation and oath according to the law of medicine, but to none others. I will follow that system of regimen which, according to my ability and judgment, I consider for the benefit of my patients, and abstain from whatever is deleterious and mischievous. I will give no deadly medicine to any one if asked, nor suggest any such counsel; and in like manner I will not give a woman a pessary to produce abortion. With purity and with holiness I will pass my life and practice my Art. I will not cut persons laboring under the stone, but will leave this to be done by men who are practitioners of this work. Into whatever houses I enter, I will go into them for the benefit of the sick, and will abstain from every voluntary act of

Edelstein, post-Hippocratic and reflecting the opinions of the Neo-Pythagorean school), *The Law,* and *The Physician* deal entirely with the professional attitude and the ethical obligations of the physician. They reflect the vital role played by apprenticeship as the basis of medical education. The *Aphorisms* discusses all aspects of medical practice and is particularly detailed on the subject of the "critical days" in the development of a disease.

In spite of their contradictions, all the Hippocratic books have some fundamental traits in common. First, they stress the naturalistic approach, as expressed in medicine's famous Declaration of Independence, given in the first lines of *On the Sacred Disease:* "It is thus with regard to the disease called Sacred: it appears to me to be nowise more divine nor more sacred than other diseases, but has a natural cause from which it originates like other affections. Men regard its nature and cause as divine from ignorance and wonder, because it is not at all like other diseases."[2]

Secondly, most of these books put great emphasis on the value of observation of the disease process, on the practical rather than the theoretical. This concentration on observation of the disease process, instead of the disease cause, relegates speculative theories to minor importance. In the observational method of the Hippocratic physicians the method of induction gained its first triumph in science. The following quotations from the Hippocratic writings will illustrate the power of observation possessed by the Hippocratic phy-

---

mischief and corruption; and, further, from the seduction of females or males, of freemen and slaves. Whatever, in connection with my professional practice or not, in connection with it, I see or hear, in the life of men, which ought not to be spoken of abroad, I will not divulge, as reckoning that all such should be kept secret. While I continue to keep this Oath unviolated, may it be granted to me to enjoy life and the practice of the art, respected by all men, in all time! But should I trespass and violate this Oath, may the reverse be my lot! (Hippocrates, in *Works,* trans. by Francis Adams [London, 1849], Vol. I, pp. 278–80).

2 Hippocrates, "On the Sacred Disease," in *Works,* Vol. II, p. 843.

sician and the amount of empirical insight which could be gained from this method:

He [the physician] should observe thus in acute diseases: first, the countenance of the patient, if it be like those of persons in health, and more so, if like itself, for this is the best of all; whereas the most opposite to it is the worst, such as the following; a sharp nose, hollow eyes, collapsed temples; the ears cold, contracted, and their lobes turned out; the skin about the forehead being rough, distended, and parched; the color of the whole face being green, black, livid, or lead-colored. If the countenance be such at the commencement of the disease, and if this cannot be accounted for from the other symptoms, inquiry must be made whether the patient has long wanted sleep; whether his bowels have been very loose; and whether he has suffered from want of food; and if any of these causes be confessed to, the danger is to be reckoned so far less; and it becomes obvious, in the course of a day and a night, whether or not the appearance of the countenance proceeded from these causes. But if none of these be said to exist, and if the symptoms do not subside in the aforesaid time, it is to be known for certain that death is at hand.[3]

The abundant details in the following description leave no doubt that the people of Thasos were suffering from mumps:

In Thasus, about the autumnal equinox, and under the Pleiades, the rains were abundant, constant, and soft, with southerly winds; the winter southerly, the northerly winds faint, droughts; on the whole, the winter having the character of spring. The spring was southerly, cool, rains small in quantity. Summer, for the most part, cloudy, no rain, the Etesian winds, rare and small, blew in an irregular manner. The whole constitution of the seasons being thus inclined to the southerly, and with droughts early in the spring, from the preceding opposite and northerly state, ardent fevers occurred in a few instances, and these very mild, being rarely attended with hemorrhage, and never proving fatal. Swellings appeared about the ears, in many on either side, and in the greatest number on both sides, being unaccompanied by fever so as not to confine the patient to bed; in all cases they disappeared without giving trouble, neither did any of them come to suppuration, as is common in swellings from other causes. They were of a lax, large, diffused character, without inflammation or pain, and they went away

3 Hippocrates, "Prognostics," in *Works*, Vol. I, p. 235.

without any critical sign. They seized children, adults, and mostly those engaged in the exercises of the palestra and gymnasium, but seldom attacked women. Many had dry coughs without expectoration, and accompanied with hoarseness of voice. In some instances earlier, and in others later, inflammations with pain seized sometimes one of the testicles, and sometimes both; some of these cases were accompanied with fever and some not; the greatest part of these were attended with much suffering. In other respects they were free of disease, so as not to require medical assistance.[4]

Finally, here are some examples from *Aphorisms:* "Fat persons are more exposed to sudden death than the slender" (II, 713). "Those who swoon frequently, and without apparent cause, are liable to die suddenly" (congenital heart disease?) (II, 712). "Spasm supervening upon a wound is fatal" (Tetanus) (II, 737). "Spinal deformity often coexists with cough and tubercle of the lungs" (II, 760). "Diarrhea in phthisis is a mortal symptom (II, 739).[5]

Observation in the Hippocratic period was primarily based on inspection and palpation. The sense of smell was also used, and a crude kind of auscultation was practiced, as for instance in the so-called succussion, which consisted of shaking a patient and listening for fluid. The Hippocratic writings deal mainly with acute, easily identifiable diseases, such as the present-day disease entities of pneumonia, phthisis, puerperal fever, anthrax, mumps, and particularly malaria. Chronic diseases were to the Hippocratic physician only the sequel of acute diseases. Yet, though they were observed and described, few of these disease entities were named in the Hippocratic writings. They were not related to anatomical changes, and no diagnosis in the modern sense was made. Diseases were classified only into the acute and the chronic, the epidemic and the endemic. This attitude of the Hippocratic physician was not due to a lack of mental powers but was rather an expression of his fundamentally different approach. The Hippocratic physician was primarily interested,

[4] Hippocrates, "Epidemics," in *Works*, Vol. I, p. 352.
[5] Page citations refer to Hippocrates, "Aphorisms," in *Works*.

not in diagnosis, but in prognosis and treatment. His first interest was not in a disease manifested in the patient, but in the patient himself. He was concerned with the body as a whole rather than with the lesion of parts. Here, he partly transformed a shortcoming into a virtue. His knowledge was far too limited to practice diagnostics and specific treatments successfully.

This emphasis on prognosis is easily explained by the peculiar, unprotected social position of the Greek physician. He was a traveling craftsman and had to gain the public's confidence rapidly through marvelous prognoses. Since he could not afford failure, it was of the utmost importance to him to know whether or not he should accept treatment of a patient—and sometimes even whether or when he would have to leave town. There is no doubt that these social factors played a powerful role in shaping the opinions and practice of the Greek physician. It is also possible that other factors, such as the intense interest of all ancient cultures in omens, contributed to the development of his attitude.

Though the Hippocratic physician was primarily a craftsman, he nevertheless had some grounding in philosophy and rhetoric, a grounding that he needed as a background for his art. Unlike the present-day physician, surrounded by the medieval dignity of the doctor, he not only had to explain his actions to his philosophically educated upper-class patients, but also was called on to sustain in their presence discussions on his art with other physician-craftsmen or philosophers dabbling in medicine.

The treatment of the Hippocratic physician reflected his fundamental approach. It was the treatment of an individual, not of a disease, and the treatment of the whole body, not of any part of it. Treatment was based on the fundamental assumption that nature, *physis*, had a strong healing force and tendency of its own, and that the main role of the physician was to assist nature in this healing process, rather than to direct it arbitrarily. Health was a state of harmonic mixture of the humors (*eucrasia*), and disease was a state of

faulty mixture (*dyscrasia*). The disordered humors were in a
state of *apepsis,* and nature itself tried to re-establish balance through a process of *pepsis* or coction through the so-
called innate heat. This coction—which simply means "cook-
ing"—usually ended with a *crisis* on a "critical day," when
the diseased matter, the end product of coction, was eliminated. Sometimes disease petered out slowly in *lysis* instead
of *crisis.*

The main ally of the physician in assisting nature in this
process was diet. More violent means of elimination, such
as purging, vomiting, and bloodletting, were seldom used by
the Hippocratics. Only if diet failed were drugs used, and
surgery was a last resort. In spite of the generally conservative character of Hippocratic surgery, some rather daring
operations were performed, including the trepanation of the
skull and the opening of empyemas.

The humoral disturbances, which were felt to be the basic
cause of disease, were not clearly differentiated in most Hippocratic writings from difficulties of the *pneuma,* a rather
mysterious substance which in modern terms might mean
anything from oxygen to the soul. Diseases could be caused
by excesses and strains experienced by the patient, by climatic influences (the epidemic constitution), or by the bodily,
more or less inherited, constitution of the patient.

Hippocratic disease theories were clearly conditioned by
the rudimentary technology of the period. The four-humor
physiology was not even a chemical theory but, as the word
"coction" suggests, a physiology derived from observations
in the kitchen. The overwhelming influence on the body attributed to climate and weather indicates the occupational
views of the navigator, so dependent on weather, and the
agriculturist, to whom the human body is like a field exposed
to the vagaries of the seasons.

High ethical ideals pervade all the Hippocratic writings.
The Hippocratic author of *Epidemics,* for instance, provides
a rare example of scientific honesty in reporting forty-two

cases out of which twenty-five were fatal. Kindness ("Where is love of men there is also love of the art") and dignity are emphasized, as well as the more technical virtues of cleanliness and dexterity. Even more than other parts of the Hippocratic writings, the ethical precepts show a deep wisdom. The callous-sounding injunctions not to treat incurables must be understood in the light of the times. Because of the Hippocratic physician's unstable professional position and inferior social status, it was paramount that he avoid the stigma of failure. From a craftsman's point of view this refusal to repair the irreparable is ethical.

Aristotle (384–322 B.C.), the great philosopher and biologist of the time immediately after the Hippocratic period, had considerable influence on medicine, especially during the late Middle Ages and the Renaissance, less through his encyclopedic attempts to describe the whole of nature and man, than through certain basic principles: everything tends from matter, from the potential to form, the actual, and the enteloechy. Every creation has a goal. Man is the purpose of nature. All being is motion in time and space. The most perfect movement is the circle. Aristotle's influence was not always good, neither in general nor in particular cases; teleology is often misleading. The work of his pupil Theophrastus (370–286 B.C.), the "father of botany," is rather part of the history of science than of the history of medicine, since Theophrastus' magnificent writings on botany are not particularly concerned with the pharmacological properties of the plants described.

Chapter 7

GREEK MEDICINE: ALEXANDRIA
AND ROME

There is a three-hundred-year gap in the documentation
of Greek medicine between the *Corpus Hippocraticum* and
the works of the Roman encyclopedist Celsus, who lived
about A.D. 30. It is only the quotations in Celsus and in later
Greek medical authors that reveal the numerous changes of
the post-Hippocratic period. When at last Greek medicine
reappears in the pages of Celsus, it has lost much of its original simplicity and has produced many idle speculations; but
it has also achieved much real progress.

The fact that very little original medical writing has survived between the *Corpus Hippocraticum* and Galen, both
humoralists, probably accounts for the myth that Greek medicine was consistently humoralistic throughout the thousand
years of its creative existence. Even on the basis of the
limited information available, it is safe to say that this was
not true. One school followed another. Centers shifted
continuously. The diagram on page 68 illustrates the great
variety of approaches developed. All approaches listed on
the right side of the central dotted line in this diagram were
nonhumoralistic. It was only after Galen, who became the
authoritative representative of the Greek legacy, that the
humoral theory of disease began its almost undisputed reign,
which lasted about fifteen hundred years.

The immediate followers of Hippocrates have been called
"Dogmatists," a name which implies sterile imitation of the
great example. This description certainly does not hold true
for the best of the Dogmatists, such as Diocles of Carystus

and Praxagoras of Cos. Diocles made extensive studies of anatomy, though these did not deter him from regarding the heart as the central organ of the body and the seat of mental disease. Praxagoras lived about 340 B.C. and seems to have been the first Greek physician to make a closer study of the changes of the pulse in disease.

In the third century B.C. the center of Greek civilization and medicine shifted from the old Greek settlements toward the new Egyptian city of Alexandria. This city was named after the Macedonian king, Alexander the Great, who carried Greek civilization to the limits of the then known world. In the strange cultural melting pot of Alexandria, Greek science produced some of its greatest achievements, and, conversely, Oriental mysticism gained greater influence on Greek thinking. The decline in the fields of art and philosophy was unmistakable in Alexandria. On the other hand a utilitarian attitude brought about great progress in the sciences—astronomy, geography, and the mathematics of Euclid and Archimedes—and particularly in the field of technology, as illustrated by the mechanics of Hero and Archimedes. Progress in technology led to an unavoidable trend toward specialization. The wonderful libraries of Alexandria and its museum, a combination of boarding house for scholars and university, offered unique possibilities for a luxuriant growth of scholarship. The early Alexandrian period is the only period in the history of Greek medicine where dissection was legalized. This produced the most gratifying results for anatomical and surgical knowledge.

The names of Herophilus and Erasistratus have become symbols of the Alexandrian school of the early period. Herophilus of Chalcedon (about 300 B.C.) made important contributions to all fields of anatomy. He gave good descriptions of the eye, the brain, the vessels of the body, the duodenum (named by him), and the male and female genital organs. He observed that sensor and motor paralysis are not necessarily simultaneous in a body region. He tried to make pulse observations more objective and counted the pulse with

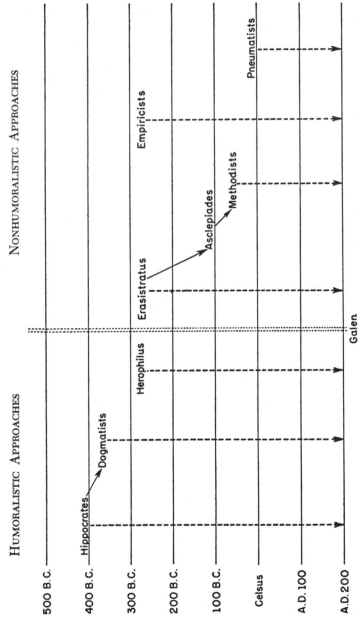

Chronological table of Greek medical sects. The productive years of Greek medicine evolved a great variety of approaches, most of which persisted for a considerable length of time. The humoral theory was by no means the prevailing approach before the time of Galen.

a water clock. Originally a follower of Hippocrates, Herophilus came under the influence of sceptic philosophy. This prevented him from radically breaking with humoralism and from drawing far-reaching conclusions from his experiments. As a therapist he had more confidence in drugs, "the hands of the Gods," and in venesection than the Hippocratic school. He was strongly interested in surgery and obstetrics. His medical thinking is well summarized in his famous aphorism: "The best physician is the one who is able to differentiate the possible and the impossible."

None of the sixty-two books of Erasistratus of Cos (born about 330 B.C. and reported to have committed suicide because of incurable cancer about 250 B.C.) has survived. Erasistratus, too, was a great anatomist. He noted the existence of separate sensory and motor nerves and gave many details on the anatomy of the brain and cerebellum, the heart, and the veins and arteries. He tried to approach the riddle of metabolism by weighing the intake and excrement of fowls and noting the loss of matter through "insensible perspiration." Erasistratus made the first observations in pathological anatomy. He noted the hardening of the liver in ascites and regarded the former as a cause of the latter.

Erasistratus accepted the consequences of his anatomical research; he gave up Hippocratic humoral pathology in favor of a pathology of solids. He regarded atoms as the essential body elements. These atoms, he reasoned, were vitalized by external air (*pneuma*) circulating through the arteries. He had a purely mechanistic concept of digestion, and regarded disease as primarily caused by a local plethora interfering with the circulation of the *pneuma*. Solidistic pathology is thus an Alexandrian invention. In the following centuries it shared the fate of the heliocentric system of the Alexandrian Aristarchus. As a therapist, Erasistratus was on the whole opposed to bleeding and polypharmacy. Both Herophilus and Erasistratus were the founders of schools which lasted until the second century A.D.

Toward the end of the third century B.C. a third medical group developed in Alexandria. They called themselves Empiricists. Philinos of Cos (about 250 B.C.), Serapion of Alexandria (about 220 B.C.), and Glaucias of Tarus (about 170 B.C.) were the pioneers in this movement. Heraclides of Tarus, who lived at the beginning of the first century B.C., was perhaps the foremost of the Empiricists. His experiments with drugs made valuable contributions to the field of pharmacy.

The Empiricists were essentially in revolt against the philosophical speculations and scientific experiments which seemed to them irrelevant to medical practice. They reduced medical lore to their own observations, complemented by the observations of older authors. Their treatments were based on analogies. This Empiricist reaction was only the first of many similar movements in the history of medicine. These movements, psychologically easy to understand but sooner or later coming to a dead end because of their limited outlook, have usually made real contributions to medicine. Thus Empiricism, while not a dynamic factor in the future development of medicine, enriched specific fields, particularly symptomatology, pharmacology, and surgery. In connection with solidism and the progress of physics, anatomy, and technology, surgery advanced greatly in Alexandria until Roman times. We hear now, among other things, of the ligature being used as a hemostatic, of operations of goiter, hernia, cataract, and tonsils, and of plastic operations. At Alexandria, surgery seems to have begun its separation from internal medicine.

During the same period many of the numerous small tyrants of the Middle East turned to medical research. Their interest was more personal than scientific, and the object of their preoccupation was a special branch of the drug family —the poisons. Poisons have fallen out of fashion in modern times because science has made their detection easy. But they have been powerful allies of the ambitious throughout history. Knowledge of poisons and their antidotes was very important for a dictator. The best known of these royal amateur toxicologists was King Mithridates of Pontus (120–63 B.C.), the last powerful enemy of the Romans in the Near East. A very common antidote of late antiquity and the Middle Ages was named after him. In his experiments with ducks he supposedly hit upon the idea that one could immunize against poisons through repeated application of small doses.

The stage for the last great drama of Greek medicine is set in Rome. Ever since the third century B.C. Greek physicians, freemen, and slaves had been drifting into Rome. At first the Romans energetically opposed the use of foreign physicians, partly out of a feeling of national pride and partly because the professional and ethical standards of the new arrivals were often rather low. But accomplishment by the Romans themselves in the field of medicine was conspicuously absent. In the long run Greek medicine was bound to triumph in Rome.

The definite establishment of Greek medicine in Rome was brought about by the strong personality of Asclepiades, a Greek physician from Asia Minor, born in the year 124 B.C. The influence of Erasistratus on Asclepiades' medical thinking is unmistakable. Asclepiades was opposed to empiricism and to humorism. His pathology was solidistic and atomistic. He thought that the cause of disease was a mechanical disturbance of the movement of atoms through the pores of the body. Like Erasistratus, he did not believe in the automatically beneficial effect of nature's actions and structures. He found harsh words for the passive attitude of the Hippocratic physician, whose practice he called a long waiting for death, and he opposed the lore of critical days. According to Asclepiades the *pneuma* brought animation into the whole body. Asclepiades studied mental disease and made decerebration experiments. The therapeutic methods of Asclepiades, popularized by the slogan *cito, tuto, jucunde* (fast, safe, and agreeable), were far less energetic than one might suppose from his theories. His fight against too active treatments made him a great reformer of therapeutics. He was opposed to blood-letting and purging, and relied primarily on diet, baths, and carefully developed gymnastics. His popularity as a physician can easily be understood from the fact that one of his preferred dietetic remedies was wine. Asclepiades recommended tracheotomy in case of obstruction of the upper respiratory passages.

Asclepiades opened the way for a new medical sect, the Methodist, founded by Themison of Laodicea about 50 B.C. The Methodists, as the name implies, reduced the theory of medicine and therapeutics to a few very simple methods. Disease was caused either by *status strictus,* a narrowing of the internal pores, or by *status laxus,* an excessive relaxation of the pores. Treatment, therefore, was concerned only with overcoming excessive contraction or excessive relaxation. Such oversimplified disease theories have been influential in medicine at least up to the beginning of the last century. The Roman encyclopedist Celsus attributed the genesis of Methodism to the necessity of treating large numbers of patients on the big slave plantations with a minimum of effort. The Roman inclination toward formalism may also have been a formative element in Methodism. The most famous member of the Methodist school was Soranus of Ephesus (about A.D. 100), who must have been a great physician. He is remembered for his accomplishments in gynecology and obstetrics.

Some medical books by Soranus have survived under the name of a Latin translator, Caelius Aurelianus. They show Soranus as a man of sufficient intelligence to abandon the principles of Methodism when clinical necessities demanded it. The work which now bears the name of Caelius Aurelianus is the only surviving ancient text to contain a full and orderly discussion of mental disease, of which the ancients knew primarily three: melancholy, mania, and phrenitis, the fever delirium which was apparently more prevalent then because of the frequency of fevers. The names given to mental diseases indicate a purely somatic approach. Hysteria (disease of the uterus) and hypochondria (disease below the diaphragm) were not even classified as mental diseases. The ancient physicians, proud of their emancipation from supernaturalistic beliefs, regarded mental disease as a bodily phenomenon and treated it accordingly, generally by some sort of evacuation. Their considerable use of psychotherapeutic methods was purely empirical and somewhat accidental.

The last Greek school of medicine was that of the Pneumatists. Pneumatism was undoubtedly strongly influenced by the Stoic philosophy, and its disease theory was based on the vagaries of the *pneuma*. The founder of the school was Athenaeus of Attalia (first century A.D.). Pneumatism soon developed into Eclecticism, which gradually became the prevailing attitude of the physicians of late antiquity. One of the outstanding members of the Pneumatic school was Archigenes (about A.D. 100), whose writings reveal an exceptional skill in surgery, including the techniques of amputation and ligature. These writings also contain a highly developed drug lore and make a praiseworthy attempt to differentiate between primary and secondary phenomena of disease. It is immaterial whether the fragmentary writings of Aretaeus (about A.D. 150), of whom nothing is known but his name, are original or mere copies of the writings of Archigenes. Whoever the author was, the extraordinary clinical descriptions of diabetes, tetanus, diphtheria, and leprosy show clearly that the clinical genius of the Greeks was still as alive and powerful in the second century A.D. as it had been in the sixth century B.C. The description of diabetes is a good example:

DIABETES is a strange affection, not very frequent among men, being a melting of the flesh and limbs into urine. Its cause is of a cold and humid nature, as in dropsy. The course is the common one, namely, the kidneys and bladder; for the patients never stop making water, but the flow is incessant, as if from the opening aqueducts. The nature of the disease, then, is chronic, and it takes a long period to form; but the patient is short-lived, if the constitution of the disease be completely established; for the melting is rapid, the death speedy. Moreover, life is disgusting and painful, thirst unquenchable; excessive drinking, which, however, is disproportionate to the large quantity of urine, for more urine is passed; and one cannot stop them either from drinking or making water. Or if for a time they abstain from drinking, their mouth becomes parched and their body dry; the viscera seem as if scorched up; they are affected with nausea, restlessness, and a burning thirst; and at no distant term they expire. Thirst, as if scorched up with fire. But by what method could they be restrained from making water? Or how can shame become more potent than pain?[1]

Medicine remained in Greek hands throughout antiquity. The Romans, with their essentially utilitarian approach, did great things in the fields of law, government, warfare, and architecture, but they never developed any original talent in philosophy, art, or science. Latin medical works were essentially compilations. The most famous work is that of Celsus, a Roman gentleman to whom medical historians owe a great debt, especially for his preservation of information about the Alexandrian physicians. Celsus was largely influenced by Hippocratic thought, but his descriptions of surgical practice reflect a much higher level of accomplishment, including the use of the ligature and performance of the cataract operation. The richness of Celsus in dermatological details is still reflected in present-day dermatological nomenclature. Since he was only a compiler, Celsus was never mentioned by ancient physicians, and he became famous only during the Renaissance, about fifteen hundred years after his death. The same holds true for another compiler, Pliny the Elder (A.D. 23–79), whose uncritical collection of facts and fancies deeply impressed the Renaissance and later physicians. The Roman Scribonius Largus (about A.D. 47) left a collection of prescriptions. A comparison of the work of Scribonius with that of the Greek army surgeon Dioscorides, who served under Nero (A.D. 54–68), illustrates the great difference in quality between Greek and Latin medical writings. Dioscorides is the father of our *materia medica*. He described over 600 medicinal plants and was a

[1] *The Extant Works of Aretaeus,* trans. by Francis Adams (London, 1856), p. 338.

superb pharmacognosist. As a therapist, he naively believed in all kinds of panaceas. The Greek physician Rufus of Ephesus (about A.D. 100) cannot be classed with any medical sect or school, but he is important for his anatomy, for his pulse lore, and for his clinical details on cancer and plague.

The end of the creative period of Greek medicine is marked by Galen of Pergamum (A.D. 130–201), probably the greatest of Greek physicians after Hippocrates. The multiplicity of sects and approaches had resulted in a deep desire for synthesis. It was Galen who best satisfied this need. While very little is known about the personal life of Hippocrates, that of Galen is well documented. His father was an architect. Galen was born in 130 in Pergamum in Asia Minor, the site of a famous temple of Asclepius. For nine years Galen studied medicine and philosophy in Smyrna, Corinth, and Alexandria. Then he returned to his home town to become physician to the gladiators. After four years he left for Rome where he soon gained great fame as a practitioner, lecturer, and experimenter. A "plague" caused him to flee from Rome for a time, behavior which was regarded as perfectly ethical up to the eighteenth century. He soon returned to become the body physician of the Emperor-philosopher Marcus Aurelius. Galen died in 201. An extremely fertile author, he wrote at least a hundred treatises. His surviving works fill no less than twenty-two volumes.

Galen's wordy, aggressive, and self-laudatory writings do not reveal a very attractive personality. There is also a widespread prejudice against Galen because of the very paralyzing role played by his writings in the medicine of the Middle Ages and early modern times. Yet for the latter phenomenon, at least, it was certainly not he who was responsible, but the conservatism and authoritarianism of the period. The easily aroused prejudices against Galen should not blind the reader to the fact that he was far more than a compiler. Galen was a first-rate anatomist and physiologist, and with him medicine took a great step forward. In spite of his frequent declarations of reverence for Hippocrates,

Galen was no Hippocratist. In the Hippocratic writings medicine remained essentially an art. With Galen it became a science, often a deficient science, but a science none the less.

Galen was a great dissector and made great advances in the knowledge of muscles and bones, though less so in that of vessels, nerves, and viscera. His knowledge was chiefly gained through the dissection of monkeys and pigs (he once dissected an elephant, but apparently never a human) and was therefore of only limited validity as far as human anatomy was concerned. Nevertheless, he eliminated such basic, time-honored errors as the belief that the heart was the origin of nerves and the brain of blood vessels. He described the brain and its ventricles and placed the medulla as a part of the brain. He showed the difference between sensory and motor nerves, which he called soft and hard nerves. Galen was even more outstanding as an experimental physiologist. He established the function of the recurrent nerve by cutting it and producing loss of voice. He obtained arrest of respiration by cutting the medulla. His experiments on the spinal cord produced cross-lesions. By tying the femoral arteries he showed that arteries contained blood, and by tying the ureters he demonstrated that urine is produced in the kidney, not in the bladder as had been falsely assumed. His experimental animals were monkeys, pigs, and dogs.

On the other hand, Galen was no modern scientist. He did not limit himself to conclusions derived from dissections and experiments, but built up a wide speculative system of physiology. This system is most fully expounded in his treatises *On the Faculties* and *On the Use of the Parts*. His most famous physiological theory is that of the blood flow, which dominated medicine up to the time of Harvey (see accompanying diagram). According to this theory, the nutritive substances were carried from the intestines into the liver, where the "natural spirits" transformed them into blood. Part of this blood flowed by way of the veins directly into the periphery. The rest went into the right ventricle of the heart, from which a small part moved into the lung, while the

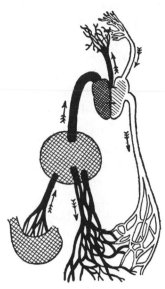

Galen's theory of blood movement and formation of the spirits. According-ing to Galen, the blood reached the periphery through the veins (most of it departing from the liver) as well as through the arteries (departing from the heart). Little blood went to the lungs from the right ventricle of the heart; he thought most of the blood passed from the right to the left ventricle through "pores" in the intraventricular septum.

remainder passed through pores in the septum into the left ventricle. In the heart the blood was endowed with "vital spirits" (entering through the lung) and carried through the arteries into the periphery again. Some of the blood reached the brain, where the "animal spirits" were developed and dispersed into the body through the nerves.

Galen was bolstered in his speculations by the teleological beliefs—nature does nothing in vain—which he had inherited from Aristotle. He was a monotheist, and Moses and Christ are mentioned in his writings. He believed that the creator had endowed every organ with a special purpose from which its function could be deduced. Galen's influence interrupted the nonteleological tradition of atomists such as Asclepiades and Anaxagoras, who regarded the body as an accidental aggregation of atoms, and function as conditioning form.

Galen was a great dialectician, never at a loss to find by reason an answer to every question.

Galen's pathology was primarily the humoral pathology of some of the Hippocratic writers and of Aristotle. But as an Eclectic he occasionally used the notion of *pneuma,* dear to the Stoic philosophers, and the *strictum* and *laxum* of the Methodists, when these fitted his purposes. The "critical days" played a great role in Galen's pathology, and the prevailing acute diseases, pneumonia, typhoid fever, and malaria, supported such a belief. Galen was interested in diagnosis as well as prognosis. In *On the Affected Parts* he made an important step toward local pathology when he stated that a function is never impaired without the part governing the function being affected. He quoted with great pride his diagnosis of a broken vertebra on the basis of an insensibility in the fourth and fifth fingers of a man who had fallen on his back. Galen tried to distinguish between abdominal pain caused by kidney stones and pain caused by an affection of the intestines. He also tried to differentiate between hemoptoe, the spitting of blood, and hematemesis, the vomiting of blood. Measurement of the pulse and inspection of the urine played a great role in his diagnostics. In spite of his contributions to anatomy and to the localization of disease, Galen's pathology remained essentially humoral and therefore uncongenial to localistic and anatomical thought.

Galen's therapeutics were schematic, following a *methodus.* For instance, "cold" remedies were used against "hot" diseases and vice versa. Unlike the therapeutics of the Hippocratics, his therapeutics were mainly active. He was addicted to polypharmacy; sometimes as many as twenty-five drugs were used in one prescription, and such complicated prescriptions were henceforth called Galenics. He used bleeding and evacuation frequently. He prescribed climatic treatment for tuberculosis. Galen was very much concerned with hygiene and stated in a rather modern fashion that prevention is preferable to treatment.

He had developed into a good surgeon and physiotherapist while treating gladiators. Indicative of the beginning of the cleavage between surgery and medicine was the fact that Galen no longer practiced surgery to any great extent after coming to Rome. In that slave-holding society, manual labor was considered beneath the dignity of a gentleman, and surgery was regarded as a form of manual labor.

Galen subscribed to the theory of "laudable pus," which held that every wound produced pus normally in the process of healing. As a result, this theory became a tradition which up to the nineteenth century prevented aseptic treatment of wounds. Galen himself was far less dogmatic about the matter and obviously was able to heal tendons *per primam intentionem* (immediately, before pus formation).

Our picture of Galen has been distorted by the misuse which was later made of his writings, a misuse for which he cannot be held responsible. It is true that his systematism and his teleology, which made him so dear to the Middle Ages, are uncongenial to the modern mind, as are his continuous bitter denunciations of his contemporaries, justified though they sometimes may have been. It is only fair to state that his system was based, not on reason alone, but on reason and experience. Galen himself was never a blind traditionalist but submitted tradition to experience and experiment. His ability to see problems was extraordinary. And Galen was, beyond any doubt, the greatest medical experimentalist, not only of his time, but of any time preceding the seventeenth century.

While this short survey has had to concentrate on the clinical knowledge and theories of Greek medicine in Rome, some social aspects of medicine in Rome should at least be mentioned. There were sickness insurance associations and medical societies in Rome; there was an increasing tendency toward specialization and the state employment of physicians; and, toward the end, mystical healing cults grew increasingly popular. All these phenomena of the increasingly complex and decadent Roman society have a rather modern ring.

The greatest medical contribution of the Romans was an indirect one. Inspired by their Etruscan predecessors, they built aqueducts, sewage systems, and bathing installations of unequaled magnificence, not only in Europe, but everywhere they went. It was in connection with building activities that three Roman authors, the agriculturists Varro (116–27 B.C.) and Columella (first century A.D.), and Vitruvius, the great architect of Emperor Augustus, advanced the bold hypothesis that malarial fever was produced by small animals or insects coming out of the swamps. Roman architects accepted this hypothesis and devised building techniques to prevent these invasions, thus considerably increasing general health and well-being.

Chapter 8

MEDIEVAL MEDICINE

While Greek medicine, very roughly speaking, covers the millennium from 500 B.C. to A.D. 500, the medicine of the next millennium, between A.D. 500 and 1500, can be characterized as medieval medicine. The problem that faced the Middle Ages in medicine, as in so many other fields, was to weld together the pagan traditions of the invading barbarians with the classical traditions of the defunct Empire and the Christian religion which the barbarians had adopted from those they conquered. Medieval medicine shows elements from all three sources in varying degrees.

Greek medicine had been sterile since the time of Galen. The "medieval" custom of merely compiling and interpreting the classical texts started long before the Middle Ages proper. Only the last of the great Greek compilers can be mentioned here, all of them probably Christians and living in Byzantium: Oribasius (325–403), Aetius of Amida (sixth century), Alexander of Tralles (sixth century), and Paulus of Aegina (625–690). But even these compilations were still far too extensive and too complicated for the simple tastes and practices of the early medieval world, and they were couched in a language which was not understood in large parts of that world. Early medieval medical texts are much simpler and poorer compilations, though taken from Greek sources. They consist mainly of lists of drugs. Their authors, primarily churchmen, all used the Latin language. While Greek had been the medical language for the last millennium, Latin was to become the language of medical texts for the next thirteen hundred years.

It is not the mere presence of supernaturalistic beliefs as such that differentiates the early medieval medical texts. Late antiquity had already been corrupted to a large extent by magic and superstition. But the supernaturalism of the Middle Ages was usually drawn from pagan and Christian sources quite separate from those used in late antiquity. The early medical compilations were often but an incidental part of works on more general subjects. Early medical compilers of the Middle Ages were Marcellus of Bordeaux (about A.D. 400), Isidore of Sevilla (A.D. 570–636), the Venerable Bede (A.D. 674–735), and the Abbott Hrabanus Maurus of Fulda (A.D. 780–856).

Medieval medicine can be subdivided into two periods. The first, covering the so-called Dark Ages, is usually called the period of monastic medicine. Monks played a predominant role in the practice of medicine and in the composition of medical texts, though there were of course still lay doctors, especially in Italy and Gaul. The numerous Jews who replaced the Greeks of antiquity as the court physicians of the Middle Ages, at the courts of lay princes as well as of the princes of the church, were certainly no churchmen. Still, after the great plague which ravaged Europe during the reign of the Byzantine Emperor Justinian (543), and after the replacement of the semibarbarian Lombards in Italy by the fully barbarian Goths (568), monasteries were left to an increasing extent as the last refuges of learning. Medicine was gradually returning to the priests. The hands of time had been turned back a thousand years in the general breakdown of civilization.

The cloister of Monte Cassino, founded in 529 and destroyed in 1944, is a symbol of the medical development of the monks. The Roman statesman Cassiodorus (480–573), who retired to this cloister, had left to its library summaries of Galen, Oribasius, and Alexander of Tralles. More monasteries were founded in the outlying districts of Spain, France, Ireland, and Germany during the following centuries. Toward the end of the Dark Ages the "cathedral" schools, such as that at Chartres about A.D. 1000, became increasingly important as centers of learning in general and of medical learning in particular.

The importance of this monastic medicine should not be overestimated. The writings of the monks were primarily of translations. They were practical treatises helpful in maintaining cloister infirmaries and herb gardens. The writings of Abbott Strabo of Reichenau in the ninth century reflect the more practical aspects of monastic medicine. However, medical activity was for the monks only an accessory to their sacred mission, as indicated by the fact that the library of the cloister of St. Gall in Switzerland had in the ninth century only six medical books as contrasted with a thousand books on theology. Yet, with all their shortcomings, these monks performed one very important service. They maintained the continuity of Western medicine and brought about some amalgamation of the scientific point of view with that of Christianity.

Despite the work of some monks in the service of medicine, early Christianity as a whole had little use for it. This is evidenced as late as the sixth century in the writings of Pope Gregory and St. Gregory of Tours. They emphasized interest in the soul as opposed to concern for bodily ills. Christianity originally held its own theory of disease; disease was either punishment for sins, possession by the devil, or the result of witchcraft. It also had its own therapeutic methods—namely, prayer, penitence, and the assistance of saints. Every cure, under these circumstances, was basically regarded as a miracle.

Monk doctors such as Hrabanus Maurus and Strabo did not deny the fundamental connections between sin and disease; rather, they sought a compromise in their approach to medicine. This compromise is best reflected in the teaching of St. Hildegard of Bingen, a twelfth-century abbess. She argued that it was important to strengthen the sick body physically so that it could withstand more easily the attacks of the devil and his assistants.

The barbarian legacy is very obvious in the magic elements of such writings as the Anglo-Saxon leech books of the tenth century. Even the therapeutic writings of St. Hildegard differ from Cherokee curing spells mainly in the substitution of the names of saints for those of nature spirits. Still, this belief in magic was nothing new or particularly medieval. It was already active in late antiquity, and it must be admitted that the church did a great deal at first to purge this kind of magic. As Thorndike has stated in his great work on magic and science in the Middle Ages, magic was more prevalent in the late than in the early Middle Ages. Its influence increased simultaneously with the growth of scientific knowledge.

The period of monastic medicine was officially closed when the Council of Clermont in 1130 forbade the practice of medicine to monks as being too disruptive an occupation for an orderly life in monastic sequestration. Medicine did not thereby become a layman's occupation. Instead it fell into the hands of the secular clergy. The monastic period was in any case approaching its end for another reason.

A new force which was to change the direction of medicine was the impact of Arab science on the Western world. This impact was felt in many fields besides medicine. The adoption of Arabic numerals and of such Arabic terms as "alcohol" and "algebra" indicates the widespread nature of the influence. Because of the preponderant influence of Arab authors on Western medicine during this period, it might appropriately be styled the age of Arabistic medicine. In practice, however, the medicine of this period is generally referred to as Scholastic medicine, since it was taught, not in cloisters, but in schools—the newly founded universities. These grew in the new or revived cities during the late Middle Ages.

Before Scholastic medicine is discussed, a brief look should be taken at the Arabs and their medicine. The Arabs, like the Franks, Saxons, and Normans, were barbarians who assimilated the legacy of the Greeks together with a new world religion. But the Arabs' ability to assimilate was apparently more highly developed, and the whole process was for them easier and speedier than for the Western barbarians. Between Mohammed's flight from Mecca (A.D. 622) and the appearance of the Arabs at the banks of the Loire in France (A.D. 737), hardly more than a century had passed. In that time Islam had conquered Arabia, the Near East, North Africa, and Spain. And in the clash between Western Christianity and the Arabs in the Crusades (1096–1272), the Arabs appear as by far the more civilized representatives of the medieval world.

Knowledge of the Greek legacy, in medicine as in other fields, came to the Arabs through Christian sectarians who were driven out of the Byzantine Empire, and who translated Greek authors into Semitic languages, first Syriac or Hebrew and later Arabic. The most famous school of such sectarian translators was that of the Nestorians in Gondeshapur, a Persian city flourishing in the sixth century. By the tenth century all essential Greek medical writings had been translated in Damascus (707), Cairo (874), and Bagdad (918). By that time the Arabs had progressed from merely translating Greek material to the development of their own classical medical literature.

The first great Arab medical writer was Rhazes or Al Rhazi (860–932), a Persian by birth. His famous treatise on smallpox and measles, the first clear medical study of smallpox, shows that he was not a mere compiler but an excellent clinician. Another proof of his originality is his experiments on monkeys with mercury. But it is typical of the general attitude of the times that even this most observation-minded of the Arab writers said that a thousand books were better than a thousand years of observation. Probably the most influential Arab writer was another Persian, Avicenna or Ibn Sina (980–1063), whose *Canon,* an encyclopedia of medicine, was the leading medical textbook of the Western and Eastern world for hundreds of years. Of the other early Arab medical writers mention should be made of Isaac Judaeus

(850–950), who dealt primarily with dietetics and uroscopy.

A second center of classical Arabic medicine developed in the Arab kingdoms of Spain. The fact that the leaders of this group were Jews shows that in regard to tolerance Islam was far superior to medieval Christianity. Abulcasim (1013–1106) was the only great surgeon among the Arabs. Avenzoar (died 1162) showed an astonishing independence of Galen and described the itch mite, the existence of which was definitely established in Western medicine only in the nineteenth century. Averroes (1126–1198) and Moses Maimonides (1135–1204), who had to flee from Spain to Egypt, were philosophers as well as medical men. Maimonides, the most famous Jewish physician of the Middle Ages, is, as a matter of fact, far more original as a philosopher than in medicine, where he was just another orthodox Galenist. The Jews were the leaders in medieval medicine because the main problem of this medical period was the preservation of the Greek legacy, and they were the best custodians of this tradition. In contrast, in the nineteenth century, their preeminent role was not based on any tradition but on their creative contributions toward dynamic medicine.

Arab medicine did not lack the traits that make Western medieval medicine so uncongenial to modern minds: the sterile adherence to classic authorities, the prevalence of astrology, the aversion to anatomical studies, the degradation of surgery, and the predilection toward cautery and laudable pus in surgery. But it was greatly superior to contemporary Western medicine in its far more complete knowledge of the Greeks, in its extensive drug lore, and in its development of medical hospitals. The victory of Arab medicine, which had always been Galenist, meant the disappearance of Methodist traditions which had still survived there in the West (Soranus). This creative period of Arab medicine came to an end when the early tolerance of the Arabs was submerged by the influence of a fanatic Islamic clergy.

It was by way of a long detour through the Near East and North Africa that Greek medical lore returned to Western culture, the Arabs acting as intermediaries. The two outstanding translators of classical material from Arabic into Latin were Constantinus Africanus (1020–1087), who worked at Salerno and at the cloister of Monte Cassino, and Gerard of Cremona (1140–1187), who worked in Toledo. It is noteworthy that both translators resided on the Arab-Christian frontier. It was no coincidence that Salerno, the first famous medical center of the Middle Ages, was close to Arab Sicily and that the first medically outstanding medieval university, Montpellier, was situated in southern France, near the Spanish border.

Salerno was not a clerical but a lay school. Flourishing in the twelfth century, it combined Arabism with a practical bent, and its curriculum was so excellent that it was accepted by the University of Paris. The numerous treatises emanating from this first great medieval medical school contain excellent clinical descriptions of dysentery and urogenital diseases. They also make interesting therapeutic references to the use of mercury ointments for skin diseases, iodine-containing seaweeds for goiter, soporific sponges, and intestinal suture. The famous *Regimen Sanitatis Salernitanum*, however, is probably of Toledan origin rather than from Salerno. Numerous women were reported to have been medical practitioners and teachers in Salerno.

The University of Montpellier was founded in 1181, and other outstanding medieval seats of learning date from about the same period. The University of Paris was founded in 1110, Bologna in 1113, Oxford in 1167, and Padua in 1222. The medical men in these universities were clerics. As a matter of fact, celibacy for medical men at the University of Paris was required until 1452. The universities provided an orderly medical education such as had never before existed. They set scholastic standards which dominated the future of medical education in Europe. They were truly international universities. Scholars and students from all countries could be found at each of them, and there were no language barriers since Latin was the universal language of the cultured world.

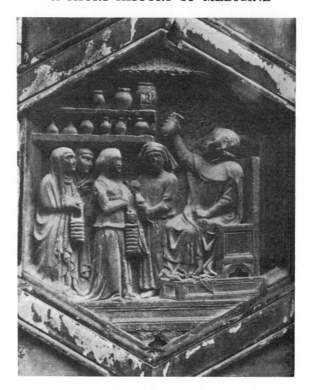

FIGURE 4. Medieval doctor examining urine.

Montpellier's greatest period falls in the thirteenth century. Famous doctors of that period, Bernard of Gordon, Gilbertus Anglicus, and John Gaddesden, were all Montpellier graduates. One graduate, Petrus Hispanus, became Pope in 1277 under the name of John XXI, the only medical man ever to have attained this dignity. Montpellier also produced at this time probably the most famous of all medieval physicians, Arnold of Villanova (1235–1312). Like many medieval physicians he was employed by princes for diplomatic missions. His reputed critical attitude toward Galen is legendary. Yet it is true that in the thirteenth century an experimental attitude was being advocated by such famous churchmen as Albertus Magnus and Roger Bacon. And perhaps it is significant that this was the century

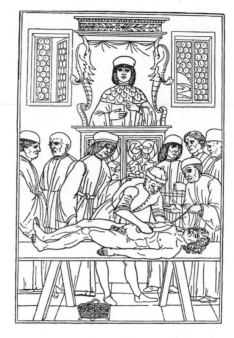

FIGURE 5. Medieval anatomy lesson.

in which the Western world began to use spectacles. Technological progress was not unknown to the Middle Ages, but it was seriously hampered by the guilds.

The Scholastic medicine of the second half of the Middle Ages was basically a mere repetition of Greek observations, theories, and prescriptions—all subjected to highly speculative discussion and interpretation. Combined with this Greek material were many elements of supernaturalism, including invocation of the numerous saints specializing in specific diseases. Authority, reasoning, and dialectics were the backbone of this medicine. As a matter of fact, in view of the corruption and contradictions in texts that had undergone so many translations and copyings, dialectial discussion was necessary if any consistent attitude was to be derived from them. For this reason outstanding medieval physicians adopted surnames indicating that they were "conciliators" (for example, Pietro d'Abano), "aggregators," or "concorders." Medieval physicians of this type were primarily philosophers, like the classical Chinese physicans, rather than scientists in the modern sense. An extensive speculative system was erected on the weakest foundation of data, as can be seen, for example, from a study of the prevailing urine and pulse lore. Uroscopy was the chief diagnostic weapon of the Medieval humoralist. Medieval philosophy in general is of real interest, especially for its progress in the field of the physical sciences; medieval art is attractive, largely perhaps, because of its complete emancipation from the classical tradition; but medieval medicine remained a complete slave to antiquity, and today it seems correspondingly unattractive. The difference between medieval medicine and modern medicine is best expressed by the verdict of Stephen d'Irsay: medieval medicine was centered, not in laboratories or hospitals, but in libraries.

Yet even such a static and stable system was susceptible to slow change. Anatomy in the fourteenth century started to become more observational and original. In that century case histories again appeared in the *concilia* of the professors of Padua and Bologna. Empirical attitudes were emphasized in the fifteenth century by men like Michele Savonarola and Nicholas of Cusa. It is no accident that advancements in medicine, as in other fields of human endeavor, came out of the Italian city republics.

Medieval medicine probably plumbed its lowest depths in the field of surgery. With the pronouncement *Ecclesia abhorret a sanguine* (the church does not shed blood), the Council of Tours (1163) effectively took surgery out of the hands of physicians, since most physicians were also clergymen. The separation of surgery and medicine, so detrimental to both disciplines, had been progressing ever since Galen's time and had been furthered by the Arab influence. During the eleventh century bloodletting was done more and more by barbers, and surgical books disappeared from the university libraries. In harmony with this movement, the Council's pronouncement gave formal sanction to a situation which was to continue for seven hundred years. Surgery was now left to barbers, bath-keepers, hangmen, sow-gelders, and mountebanks and quacks of every description.

Only in Italy and southern France, where the classical tradition did not die out entirely, did some physicians go on practicing surgery. In the writings of these outsiders are found some of the most original and worth-while medical contributions of the Middle Ages. In striking contrast to the general low standard of surgery stands the work of the four masters of Salerno and that of Hugh of Lucca and his pupil Theodoric, both of whom used the soporific sponge as a crude anesthetic and opposed the coction of wounds. Another important Italian surgeon was Saliceto of Bologna (1201–1277), who advocated the knife as opposed to Arabic cautery.

Saliceto's pupil, Lanfranc of Milan, had to leave Italy for political reasons, and thus Italian surgery was transmitted to France. Unable to join the faculty of the University of Paris because he was married, Lanfranc joined the College of St. Cosme, which had been founded in Paris in 1295. He became the body physician of the French king, Philip the Fair, and his teachings gained great authority. His contemporary, Henri de Mondeville (1260–1320), a graduate of Montpellier, was also body physician to Philip the Fair in later times. Mondeville, who made the bold statement that God did not exhaust all his creative power in making Galen, emphasized the necessity of studying anatomy and opposed the idea of coction and "laudable pus." It is regrettable that surgical tradition did not follow Mondeville instead of Guy de Chauliac (1300–1370), the body physician of the Pope of Avignon. Guy de Chauliac was an excellent surgeon who greatly improved operations for the stone and cataract, operations generally left in the hands of quacks. But unfortunately, he favored coction and the "laudable pus," and his views prevailed. Through the work of these men, however, surgery of a certain quality was kept alive until the sixteenth century, by which time the lowly barbers had themselves gathered enough strength and sophistication to enable them to contribute some of the greatest surgeons of history, including Ambroise Paré and Pierre Franco.

The anatomical illustrations of the Middle Ages are sadly similar to Chinese anatomical illustrations. The same speculative character and low quality mark them both. The church has erroneously been blamed for the low status of anatomy in this era. It has commonly been believed that dissections were forbidden by the church. This was not so. The church never forbade dissection. In fact, after the thirteenth century dissections were practiced on an increasing scale, first in Bologna (apparently originally for medicolegal reasons) and Florence, then in Montpellier, and, during the Black Death of 1349, even in Avignon at the express wish of the Pope. Nevertheless, anatomy remained unchanged, as can be seen, for instance, in the great anatomy of Mondino de Luzzi (Mundinus) of Bologna (1316). Doctors supervised dissections, but they did not actually observe what was being dissected; rather, they saw what they were supposed to see according to Galen. During these dissections the learned professor would read aloud from Galen while a lowly surgeon opened the body. Then the professor would point toward the organ and describe the five-lobed liver and other miracles of Galenic anatomy. Such was the blinding weight of tradition and authority. The two hundred years of fruitless dissection in the late Middle Ages only confirm what has already been observed among primitives, Egyptians, Babylonians, and Mexicans. The mere technique of dissection could not advance the knowledge of anatomy. What was needed was a new approach—an approach not found in the Middle Ages.

The Middle Ages are placed in time between two great epidemics: the Plague of Justinian and the Black Death. The Black Death, which in 1348 wiped out a large percentage of the European population, proved to be a powerful agent of change, affecting medicine as well as social and economic conditions. Nothing concerning plague could be found in Galen, and doctors and laymen had to rely on their own wits

in this great emergency. The Old Testament is far more con-
tagion-minded than the Greek classics, so that it is not surprising that the Middle Ages, pervaded by biblical tradition,
developed a better understanding of contagiousness than was
evidenced in late antiquity. Out of this understanding grew
the institution of quarantine as a prophylactic procedure. All
the same, the best descriptions of the Black Death were not
written by physicians, but by surgeons and laymen such as
Boccaccio. The quarantine was but one of the public health
contributions of the Middle Ages. The development of public
health measures is one of the most positive aspects of medieval medicine. Control of foods in the markets was instituted
in Germany in the twelfth century, in England in the thirteenth, and in France in the fourteenth. Control of prostitutes was instituted in London in 1165 and in Naples in 1347.

Leprosy, a rare disease among the ancients, increased
heavily after the sixth century, reached a terrifying peak in
the thirteenth century, and then mysteriously died out in
Europe. Regulations for the control of leprosy, such as isolation in leper houses, were instituted after the Council of
Lyons in 583. Another new development of the Middle Ages
was the outbreak of great epidemics of ergotism, caused by
spoiled rye. This disease was known at the time as St.
Anthony's Fire. There were also widespread epidemics of
scurvy. Psychic epidemics were especially prevalent after the
Black Death, finding expression in such acts of mass madness
as the burning of thousands of Jews, the processions of flagel-
lants, and the Children's Crusade. The dancing manias of the
fourteenth and fifteenth centuries were mainly confined to
the poor. Local epidemics of possession by the devil were
common, but medical reports on them are lacking, since they
lay in the domain of the exorcizing priest rather than the
physician.

The legal regulations of the Middle Ages covered the field
of professional organization as well as that of public health.
However medical men might feel today about the Middle
Ages, it must be admitted that they created the present title

of "doctor." With the title went a status in society, a proper education, and valuable professional organizations such as the universities, professional colleges, and guilds. While the Arab caliph Al Muqtadir had promoted medical laws as early as 931, the first medical legislation in the West was enacted by King Roger II of Sicily in 1140. It prescribed state examinations for those who wanted to practice medicine. This legislation was greatly expanded in 1224 by King Frederick II, who made provision for a nine-year curriculum, state examinations and licenses, a fee schedule, regulation of the practice of apothecaries, and control of city hygiene. Legislation of this type was adopted in Spain after 1283 and in Germany after 1347.

In any discussion of the medieval scientific doctor, recognizable in pictures wearing his fur-lined smock and holding a urine bottle, it should be remembered that these doctors formed only a very small percentage of the healing personnel. Paris, for instance, had only six such doctors in 1296, and only thirty-two in 1395. This was a proportion of one doctor for every 8,500 inhabitants. Economically these doctors were secure and did not depend on fees, being either clergymen or city-appointed. But they could not provide medical care for the mass of the population. That was left to low-class surgeons, barbers, bathkeepers, and lay healers of all descriptions. Zurich, for instance, as late as 1790, had only four academic doctors, but thirty-four barber-surgeons and eight midwives.

Perhaps the greatest medical accomplishment of the Middle Ages was the hospital. Christianity exerted in this respect the same stimulating influence that Buddhism had demonstrated earlier in India. This was not so much a reaction to certain material necessities as an expression of a new, different, more humane attitude toward the sick, which had begun in late antiquity. Although institutions rather like hospitals had existed for the benefit of slaves and soldiers under the Romans, they could not be compared in magnitude and importance to the Christian hospitals that originated under Constantine after 335. A second wave of hospital-founding had its inception—perhaps under Arab influence—in 1145 with the spread of the Holy Ghost hospitals from Montpellier. In the course of a few decades the whole of Europe was covered with a vast network of hospitals. It must of course be realized that these Christian hospitals were primarily not medical institutions but philanthropic institutions offering "hospitality" and refuge to the old, the disabled, and the homeless pilgrims. Hospitals first acquired a medical character in the institutions founded by Italian merchants under the administration of certain knightly orders in Palestine. The first provisions for regular medical care within hospitals are found in the statutes issued by the Order of St. John (founded in 1099) to its Jerusalem hospital in 1181. This transformation from charitable hospital into medical institution was greatly accelerated during the thirteenth century when administration of the hospitals was gradually taken out of the hands of the orders by city administrations.

Chapter 9

RENAISSANCE MEDICINE

The events which made up the movement known as the Renaissance marked the opening of a new period of history, the modern period. Changes had already been slowly taking place in the life of the later Middle Ages; suddenly these sped up and multiplied to an explosive extent. Any number of factors could be regarded as decisive in the formation of the new era: the large-scale introduction of gunpowder and the consequent change in warfare; the invention of printing; the discovery of the sea route to India by the Portuguese and of America by Columbus; the introduction of a money economy; or the conquest of Constantinople by the Turks in 1453 and the subsequent spread of Greek refugee scholars all over Europe.

The upheaval made itself felt in many fields. In economics, large-scale mining and banking operations were developed. In politics, peasant uprisings shook every European country. New empires arose, particularly the Spanish, which reached its peak in the sixteenth century. England started its career as a world power. The foundation of new universities in Koenigsberg, Leyden, Edinburgh, and Dublin was a sign of the increasing cultural importance of the more peripheral northern countries. In the field of religion the explosion took the form of various movements of reform and counter-reform. In the field of art the radical break with the medieval past was marked by the use of the forms of classical antiquity as a basis for the creation of new art forms. Intense individualism and a new realism characterized the ferment in all fields. Learning and science were not exempt from these changes:

Copernicus, a physician, entirely changed the concept of the universe.

Yet the times were full of contradictions. The Renaissance was not only the age of artistic creation and the cradle of modern medicine and science. It was also the age of extreme filth in cities and on persons, of the world-wide spread of diseases, of intense superstitions, and of one of the most shameful episodes in our civilization—the mass extinction of "witches." Witch-hunting was far more prevalent in the Renaissance than it had ever been before. The infamous *Witch Hammer,* a textbook for inquisitors of witches, was written in 1489. Many otherwise enlightened individuals, like Ambroise Paré and Felix Plater, believed firmly in the existence of witches.

Art was one of the first fields in which the new realism became dominant, and the new anatomical trend in medicine received strong impulses from the field of art. The thousand-year-old schematic illustrations in anatomy books were replaced at the end of the fifteenth century by new realistic designs. The relationship between artists and medical people was so close that doctors, apothecaries, and painters in Florence, one of the centers of the Renaissance, belonged to the same guild. It is impossible to describe the interrelation in detail, but the career of Leonardo da Vinci (1452–1519) illustrates it admirably. Leonardo, equally competent as artist, scientist, and engineer, and probably one of the greatest geniuses mankind has ever produced, left a great number of anatomical drawings of unprecedented quality, based on numerous dissections. But Leonardo's notes were not published until more than two hundred years after his death, and his influence during his lifetime was spread only by his limited personal contacts.

The revival of Greek learning and science, often called humanism, was made possible by the influx of Greek refugee scholars from Turkish-occupied countries. This revival gave Western scholars an opportunity to compare their corrupt translations from the Arabic with the original Greek sources. In so far as such philological research was shaking accepted authority, it had a progressive influence on the development of medicine. On the other hand, the oppressive authority of Galen was not thrown off through these efforts. It was presented in new costume only.

Of the medical philologists of the Renaissance, or medical "Humanists," one man who stands out is Leonicenus of Padua (1428–1524). His importance is not limited to the fact that he made a new and better Latin translation of Hippocrates. For in the field of botany he went beyond the narrow role of an interpreter and opened new avenues by courageously criticizing and correcting Pliny on the basis of his own observations. Leonicenus was also one of the first writers on syphilis. Since nothing could be found about this disease in Galen, its study stimulated much new thought and attracted the interest of many outstanding medical men of the period.

Botany was one of the first fields to profit from the new learning. This development was of the greatest importance to medicine at a time when therapeutics were mainly based on plant drugs. The first medical books to be printed were herbals. The groundwork for the new botany was laid in the sixteenth century by the German Protestants Otho Brunfels, Leonard Fuchs, and Hieronymus Bock (also called Tragus), and the Zurich polyhistor, Conrad Gessner. The greatest of these German Renaissance botanists was undoubtedly Valerius Cordus (1515–1544), who described five hundred new species and wrote the first modern pharmacopoeia. Remarkable advances in botany were also made by the Italians Cesalpino and Mattioli and the Frenchmen Ruellius and Pierre Belon. This period of geographical discovery and imperialist expansion also led to the founding of outstanding botanical gardens, stocked with plants brought back by travelers.

Of great importance for the further development of medicine were the new departures in clinical observation and epidemiology made in the sixteenth century. The first step was to direct criticism against the Arabs and their methods. The most famous episode in this fight was the revolt of Pierre Brissot (1478–1522) of Paris against Arab methods of bloodletting in favor of Hippocratic techniques. For this Brissot was regarded as a worse heretic than Luther, and he died in exile. The Arabic overemphasis on pulse findings and uroscopy was also widely criticized. The urinal nevertheless remained the symbol of the medical profession well up into the eighteenth century. The attack against the Arabs was often made in the name of Galen. A purified neo-Galenism was championed by men like Leonard Fuchs and Symphorien Champier. Galenism in turn was attacked by Jean Argentier (1513–1572) and his pupil Laurent Joubert (1525–1583), the dean of the Montpellier medical school, who flew the flag of a purified Hippocratism. Thus even the critical writings remained in the fold of humoralism and in the literary tradition of Scholasticism. Amatus Lusitanus (1511–1568), Zacutus Lusitanus (1575–1642), and Garcia da Orta, who were the last peaks of Jewish medieval medicine, were all orthodox Galenists. The Iberian inquisition, which persecuted them and many other physicians, rapidly terminated the short "golden age" of medicine on the Iberian peninsula.

Although most of the progressive clinicians and epidemiologists of the sixteenth century did not revolt against ancient authorities as completely as a Vesalius or a Paracelsus, still their individualization of diseases and their use of pathological anatomy marked a new departure. The posthumous book of Antonio Benivieni (1448–1502) on the hidden causes of diseases, published in Florence in 1507, was one of the first attempts to establish a close connection between autopsy findings and clinical observation during life. The work covered twenty-two case reports.

The greatest clinician of the period was the French court physician Jean Fernel (1506–1588), also a great mathematician and astronomer. Fernel's main work, *Universal Medicine*, consisted of three books: a "Physiology," a "Pathology," and a "Therapeutics." The "Physiology" and the "Pathology"

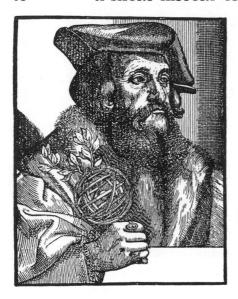

FIGURE 6. Girolamo Fracastoro.

are the earliest systematic treatises in these fields, and it was
their influence that established the subjects under these
names. Although he occasionally criticized Galen, Fernel remained faithful to the old humoral theories. However, his
frequent use of autopsies caused him to lean toward localization of disease and solidistic views. His books contain important observations of detail in the clinical field as well as in
pathological anatomy. He describes the clinical signs of influenza, the mode of infection in syphilis, which he called
lues venerea, and postmortem findings in tuberculosis, ul-
cerative endocarditis, a stone filling the renal pelvis, and a
perforated appendix. Fernel regarded gonorrhea as a separate disease, though the final separation of syphilis and
gonorrhea was accomplished only in the middle of the nineteenth century. Unlike most of the outstanding physicians of
his period, he was opposed to astrology.

Guillaume de Baillou (1538–1616) of Paris gave the first
clinical description of whooping cough, introduced the notion
of rheumatism, and revived the epidemiological theories of

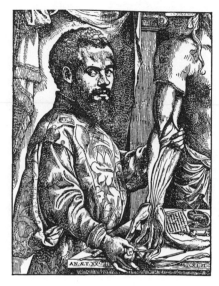

FIGURE 7. Andreas Vesalius.

Hippocrates. Other individual diseases first described during this period, and thus separated from the mass of vague "fevers" and "plagues," were the English sweating sickness, malignant tertian malaria, mountain disease, typhus, syphilis, and some of the acute exanthemata such as chickenpox and scarlet fever. The latter two diseases were isolated by Giovanni Filippo Ingrassia of Naples (1510–1580), who was also an able osteologist.

Consistent with the clinical advances of this period was the introduction of bedside teaching. This practice was introduced into medical teaching in 1543 by Montanus in Padua, one of the most important medical centers of the Renaissance. Bedside teaching was revived by Bottoni and Oddo in 1578 and carried to Leyden by their Dutch pupil, Heurne.

It is from a poem of Girolamo Fracastoro (Fracastorius) of Verona (1484–1553), physician, poet, physicist, geologist, and astrologist, that the name syphilis has been derived. The disease, then generally called French disease, Neapolitan disease, or big pox, was observed all over Europe after the un-

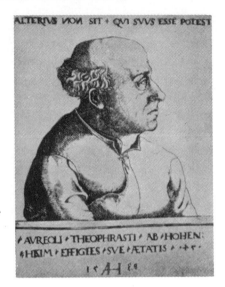

FIGURE 8.   Paracelsus.

successful siege of Naples by the French in 1495. Like many other diseases of the period it was labeled a "new disease," but only in the case of syphilis has this claim been maintained into recent times. It has been argued that the French acquired syphilis at Naples from the Spaniards, who had among them people infected through the sailors of Columbus. According to this theory the Spaniards introduced into Europe for the first time an originally American disease. The alternative view holds that syphilis was already prevalent both in Europe and in the rest of the world, but that it was only at this time that it was properly diagnosed as a result of the advance toward the individualization of disease. Much ink and emotion have been wasted on this controversy. From the evidence at hand it seems that the question cannot be resolved. Neither the literary documents nor the available bone material indicates a conclusive answer.

Fracastorius contributed to medicine far more than a new name for a loathsome disease. He also provided it with one of its most important concepts. In a book written in 1546 he presented the first consistent, scientific theory of contagious

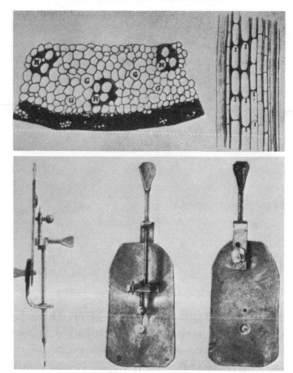

FIGURE 9. Leeuwenhoek's microscope and one of his designs.

disease, which was eventually confirmed through the discoveries of bacteriology in the nineteenth century. From his own observations and the descriptions of others he concluded that epidemic diseases were produced by small germs which had the power to multiply in the body of the patient. These germs, he believed, were spread either directly from person to person, or at a distance, or through the mediation of fomes, objects soiled with infectious material. He thought that his germs were specific, with a particular kind responsible for every epidemic disease. The varying nature of epidemics he attributed to the fact that the germs were changing in virulence. Fracastorius described and analyzed the following contagious diseases: smallpox, measles, bubonic plague,

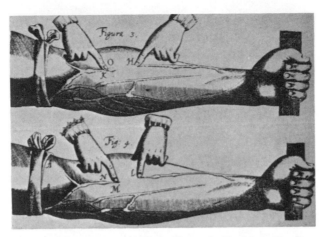

FIGURE 10. Illustration from Harvey's *De Motu Cordis*.

phthisis, leprosy, the English sweat, syphilis, typhus, and several skin diseases. He was one of the first to describe typhus. Fracastorius was fully conscious of the fact that his approach was different from the climatic approach of the ancients. His therapeutics were directly deduced from his general theory, with emphasis on the early destruction of the germ. This is an ideal which has been realized only during the last eighty years, and then only with respect to some diseases.

The efforts of the Humanists to interpret "miracles" in a rational way resulted in a greater insight into the role of psychological factors in disease. A little-understood psychological mechanism, which four hundred years ago was labeled "imagination" and which is now usually called suggestion, was recognized as being a factor in the genesis as well as in the cure of many diseases. Among the authors who studied the role of "imagination" were Cornelius Agrippa von Nettesheim, Paracelsus, Pomponatius, Pico della Mirandola, Della Porta, Cardanus, and Libavius. In connection with such studies Johann Weyer (1515–1588), a pupil of Cornelius Agrippa, made the memorable and courageous statement that the unfortunate witches were not associates of the devil but cases of mental illness. Weyer was also an able clinician, as indicated by his descriptions of the English sweat, scurvy, and the hemotakolpos, a congenital malformation of the female sex organs. Felix Plater (1536–1614) of Basle, one of the first to attempt a classification of diseases, gave particular attention to the observation and treatment of mental disease.

In no field of medical learning are the changes brought about during the Renaissance so obvious as in the field of anatomy. The weakness of medieval anatomy has already been described. In the work of Berengarius of Carpi (1470–1550), an author known for his skill in surgery and his interest in syphilis, are found the first anatomical drawings made from nature (1521). These drawings were based on more than a hundred dissections. Berengarius' reliance on dissection enabled him to describe a great number of new structures, including the sphenoid sinus, the appendix, and the hepatic circulation. Although he himself was not able to find the intraventricular pores of the heart described by Galen, he nevertheless showed himself a child of the times by accusing his forerunner, Mundinus, of not being devoted enough to the teaching of Galen.

It is the conscious abandonment of the Galenic tradition and its replacement by direct study at the dissection table that marks Andreas Vesalius (1514–1564) as the founder of modern anatomy. Vesalius is one of the greatest figures in the history of Renaissance medicine and in the history of medicine in general. Born in Brussels into a family of physicians, he studied at Louvain and Paris, and, in the truly international vein of Renaissance medicine, became professor of anatomy at Padua, the relatively liberal university in the flourishing city-state of Venice and the goal of many Northern students, at the age of twenty-three. At the age of twenty-eight he published his immortal work, *De Humani Corporis Fabrica*. In this work he showed a clear realization of the disastrous consequences of the separation of medicine from surgery and the dangers of the prevalent disdain of the academic physician for any manual activity such as dissection. He tried to re-establish the classical tradition in which such separation had been unknown. In basing his work on direct observation, he did away with such Galenic errors (resulting from the projection of pig, monkey, or dog anatomy into the human body) as the five-lobed liver, the seven-segmented sternum, the mandible consisting of two parts, the double bile duct, and the horned uterus. The excellence of Vesalius' work was enhanced by the talent of his illustrator, the Flemish artist Jan Kalkar.

Of course Vesalius could not re-create anatomy in one day; he preserved a number of errors. He was also handicapped by the relatively few samples with which he worked, which led him sometimes, as in the case of the sacrum, to take variations for normal features. Vesalius' work received the most unkind reception from the conservative chairholders, and his own teacher, Sylvius (Jacques Dubois) of Paris, gave him the nickname of Vesanus (madman). To save the authority of his beloved Galen, Sylvius thought up the ingenious argument that the human body had changed since the time of Galen. For example, he suggested that the differences in the curvature of the femur were due to the new fashion of narrow trousers. Vesalius became so disgusted with his opponents that he gave up scientific research and joined the court of the Spanish king as court physician and surgeon. In spite of his nostalgic feelings for his old occupation, he never returned to anatomy. He died on a pilgrimage to the Holy Land.

Vesalius was the greatest sixteenth century anatomist, but he was by no means the only one of importance. Although not so outspokenly opposed to Galen, Eustachius (1524–1574) was scarcely inferior to Vesalius in the description of new structures such as the eustachian tube, the suprarenals, the thoracic duct, and the abducens nerve. Vesalius' pupil and successor, Fallopius (1523–1562), gave remarkable descriptions of the female genitals and the semicircular canal. Fallopius' pupil, Fabricius ab Aquapendente (1547–1619), the teacher of William Harvey, described the valves in the veins, which later were to serve as such an important argument for

Harvey's theory of the circulation of the blood. Fabricius' interest in embryology made an equally deep impression on Harvey. Another very able anatomist was J. B. Canano, student of muscles and discoverer of the valves of the veins.

Though Vesalius gave new life to anatomy and made invaluable contributions to the development of medicine, he still clung to Galen's humoral theory. The death blow to the Galenic tradition could not come from him. It came instead from a man who made a frontal attack on the humoral theory itself. This man was Philippus Aureolus Theophrastus Bombastus von Hohenheim (1493–1541), or, as he called himself, Paracelsus.

Paracelsus reflected the violent and confused aspirations of the common man of the early sixteenth century. He represented the common man in medicine in the same way that other members of the low nobility like Saeckingen, Berlichingen, or Florian Geyer represented the common man in the peasant wars. Symbolizing his break with the past was the fact that Paracelsus was the first prominent physician to use the vernacular in his medical writings. This same vernacular was also used in the hundreds of popular medical books which flooded the market soon after the invention of the printing press.

Paracelsus was the son of a doctor. He was born in Einsiedeln, in Switzerland, and grew up in Villach, in Carinthia, where his father ministered to the workers in the mines of the famous Fuggers. He started traveling at the age of fourteen. After supposedly graduating under Leonicenus in Ferrara, he roamed over the whole of Europe for the remainder of his restless life. An attempt to settle down in Basle in 1527 failed. He is reputed to have started his activity as a professor of medicine in Basle by the rather unorthodox procedure of publicly burning the books of Galen and Avicenna. This may be a legend, but it is a legend that very well symbolizes Paracelsus' approach.

To Paracelsus there was no greater obstacle to medical progress than the traditional books. Books had to be discarded and the new physician had to return to the "book of nature." Experience, even if it was acquired by a lowly quack or "witch," was the essential element from which to build medicine. Hippocrates, the empiricist, was to him the only respectable medical authority of the past. Hippocratic and revolutionary was his own preoccupation with surgery. But thoroughly un-Hippocratic was his medieval belief that God was a direct source of medical revelation and knowledge.

Two absorbing interests for Paracelsus were alchemy and astrology. The belief in astrology was of course common among contemporary scientists and not peculiarly Paracelsian. A Fracastorius, a Copernicus, or a Kepler believed in it just as strongly as he did. Paracelsus found in astrology a substantiation for his discovery of new diseases and new drugs. He felt that, as the constellations conditioning terrestial life changed continuously, so must diseases and their treatment change.

During his youth in the Carinthian mines Paracelsus learned to be proficient in alchemy. This was the chemistry of the period, and it was as a chemist that he exerted his greatest influence on medicine. He cared little for anatomy. Most of his disease theories are of a chemical nature, the human body being regarded as a kind of alchemist's kitchen. He started a battle, which was to last for two centuries, between the new chemical "spagyric" school in medicine and the old Galenists. Paracelsus' chemical knowledge very soon showed him the unreal character of Galen's elements and humors. Unfortunately, he could not replace them with anything but the elements of his own creation, and they too were still far from reality. Alchemy was to him primarily a search for new remedies. He searched not only for new materials but for specific, causal remedies, which he called *arcana*. Thus with Paracelsus starts the search for specific remedies which is so characteristic of the modern period. Through Paracelsus' influence lead, sulfur, iron, arsenic, copper sulfate, and potassium sulfate were introduced into the pharmacopeia. The use of mercury was refined. He employed opium on a large scale in the form of laudanum. He produced ether in the course of his experiments and observed its inebriating effect on chickens.

Paracelsus justified the use of new remedies by the discovery of new diseases. He was indeed the first to have the notion of what would now be called metabolic diseases in his postulation of a group of "tartaric diseases." Among these he included gout, which he regarded as the local deposit of normally voided metabolic products. Paracelsus was the first to connect goiter and cretinism. He also wrote the first book on miners' diseases, which were dealt with very ably in the same period by Agricola (Georg Bauer of Chemnitz). His theory that diseases sprang from seeds was another early version of the germ theory. His pioneer activities in the field of psychiatry have already been mentioned.

The tragic paradox of Paracelsus' fight against the speculative philosophical system of the Galenists was that he was forced by circumstances to build another such system for himself. If Paracelsus' framework of ideas cannot easily be identified as a "system," it is not because systematic intentions were absent but only because of his utter confusion as a thinker. Paracelsus was influenced by the neoplatonic ideas of the period, which stressed intuition as opposed to the Aristotelian rationalism of the Middle Ages. It seems unnecessary to go into the details of Paracelsus' philosophy, though to him it was another pillar of his whole medical structure. It contained many bizarre beliefs. His doctrine of the signatures, which held, for instance, that a yellow plant would cure jaundice, was a magic notion paralleled in primitive medicine. He believed in a mysterious life principle which he called the *archeus*. His view of man as a microcosm reproducing the macrocosm of the universe is a current idea in Hindu philosophy. Many of these views of Paracelsus were long influential.

Paracelsus' inventions, good and bad alike, were not kindly received by the vested interests of the profession, and this often turned his commendable courage into mere coarseness and bitterness. But, in spite of his exaggerations and vulgarity, many of his criticisms of the unethical practices of the doctors and apothecaries of his time (and of all times) are justified by the evidence.

Paracelsus is one of the most contradictory figures of a contradictory age. He was more modern than most of his contemporaries in his relentless and uncompromising drive for the new and in his opposition to blind obedience to authoritarianism and books. On the other hand, he was more medieval than most of his contemporaries in his all-pervading mystic religiosity. His writings are a strange mixture of intelligent observation and mystical nonsense, of humble sincerity and boasting megalomania. One cannot help looking at this medical Dr. Faustus—who has always been strangely attractive to Germans and equally repulsive to the French—with a strange mixture of pity, disgust, and admiration. Nothing would be more erroneous than to see in him a "modern physician." Walter Pagel has rightly called him a "magus." However one may feel about Paracelsus, his work cannot be ignored. In spite of the relentless opposition of the medical faculties, in his own person he came to be a symbol of medicine in the eyes of his contemporaries, just as Boerhaave, Virchow, or Freud were to be in later years. His weight was far greater than that of such Humanists as Fernel, Fracastorius, and Vesalius. And his influence, for better or for worse, has never entirely disappeared from medicine.

The Italian Cardanus (1501–1576) resembles Paracelsus in many ways. Cardanus was a mathematician, biologist, and physician who had a stormy career and a turbulent private life. He was an illegitimate child and a gambler, and he saw his son die on the gallows. In spite of an unlimited belief in astrology, he originated such brilliant ideas as that of a special writing for the blind (invented in its modern form by Braille in 1829), and that of a special method for teaching the deaf to communicate (realized by Ponce de Leon, 1520–1584).

The Renaissance eventually saw the rebirth of surgery, and its elevation to higher levels, through the efforts of the lowly barber-surgeons. For them, the new anatomy was of immediate, great practical value. The introduction of gunpowder considerably increased the social need for the surgeon and at the same time provided surgery with a new problem that could not be solved by philological studies of the ancients. Surgical treatises written in the vernacular by the army surgeons Brunschwig (1497) and Gersdorff (1517) dealt extensively with gunshot wounds. It was also in the field of treatment of gunshot wounds that the greatest Renaissance surgeon, Ambroise Paré (1510–1590), earned his first laurels.

Born as the son of a barber-surgeon and trained as such in the provincial city of Laval, Paré came to Paris as a young man and joined the army. In 1536 at the age of twenty-six he made his first great contribution. He found that the prevailing use of boiling oil in the treatment of gunshot wounds was detrimental. We can tell this story in his own words:

Now at that time I was a fresh water souldier, I had not yet seene wounds made by gun-shot at the first dressing. It is true, I had read *Iohn de Vigo*, in the first booke of wounds in generall, the eighth chapter, that wounds made by weapons of fire did participate of Venenosity, by reason of the pouder, and for their cure commands to cauterize them with oyle of Elders scalding hot, in which should be mingled a little Treackle; and not to saile, before I would apply of the sayd oyle, knowing that such a thing might bring to the patient great paine, I was willing to know first, before I applyed it, how the other Chirurgions did for the first dressing, which was to apply the sayd oyle the hottest that was possible into the wounds, with tents and setons; insomuch that I tooke courage to doe as they did. At last I wanted oyle, and was constrained in steed thereof, to apply a digestive of egges, oyle of Roses, and Turpentine. In the night I could not sleep in quite, fearing some default in not cauterizing, that I should finde those to whom I had not used the burning oyle dead impoysoned; which made me rise very early to visit them, where beyond my expectation I found those to whom I had applyed my digestive medicine, to feel little paine, and their wounds without inflammation or tumor, having rested reasonably well in the night: the other to whom was used the sayd burning oyle I found them feverish, with great paine and tumour about the edges of their wounds. And then I resolved with my selfe never so cruelly, to burne poore men wounded with gunshot.[1]

[1] From Paré's "Apology." Quoted in F. R. Packard, *Life and Times of Ambroise Paré* (New York, 1921), pp. 160-62.

In 1545 he published his book on gunshot wounds, encouraged by old Sylvius, who showed more insight in the case of Paré than in the case of his own pupil, Vesalius. Italian surgeons like Berengario and B. Maggi also turned against the treatment of gunshot wounds with boiling oil.

Paré participated in twenty campaigns and wrote twenty books which profoundly influenced the future of surgery. One of his greatest accomplishments was the reintroduction of the ligature in 1552. In the same year, he became the first surgeon of Henry II. The ligature had been completely abandoned since antiquity and replaced, through Arab influence, by the cautery as a means of hemostasis. Paré also reintroduced the podalic version in obstetrics. It was in Paré's time that the barber-surgeons began to take obstetrics out of the hands of midwives, where it had lain for millennia. His popularity was such that in 1557 the elite surgeons of the College of St. Cosme were obliged to accept in their ranks this barber who did not even know Latin. Paré, then a court surgeon, was spared in the notorious massacre of the night of St. Bartholomew in 1572, in which so many other Protestants were assassinated. He also escaped poisoning attempts that sprang from the same pious intentions.

In 1582, in his treatise on the unicorn and the mummy, two very fashionable remedies of the period, Paré destroyed the reputation of these two fake drugs for ever. Unbroken in vigor, he fathered a son in 1583 at the age of seventy-three. Shortly before his death he showed the same courage that he had displayed throughout his life when, in the streets of besieged Paris, he admonished the Archbishop of Lyons to surrender the city to Henry IV for the sake of the poor, who were dying from starvation in great numbers.

It is hard in the age of democracy to appreciate the tremendous implications of the rise of a lowly barber to such social and scientific heights in the highly stratified society of the Renaissance world. Only the highest intellectual endowment, coupled with relentless labor and study and the greatest strength of character, could achieve such a result. The humility of the man is all the more striking; at the end of such a career he could still say: *"Je le pansais, Dieu le guérit"* (I bandaged them, but God he healeth them).

Another outstanding surgeon of the period, also coming from the lower social strata, was Pierre Franco (about 1500). A native of southern France, he had to flee to Switzerland because of his Protestant beliefs. He greatly improved operations for hernias, stones, and cataracts. Gasparo Tagliacozzi (1546–1599) of Bologna revived rhinoplasty, but he had to suffer for this meddling with the work of God even after his death when he was exhumed and buried in unconsecrated ground. England participated in the renaissance of surgery through the works of Thomas Gale (1507–1586) and William Clowes (1540–1604).

Chapter 10

MEDICINE IN THE SEVENTEENTH CENTURY

The seventeenth century occupies a unique position in the history of science. It is the century of the mathematician-philosophers Descartes, Leibnitz, and Pascal; of the physicist-astronomers Newton, Galileo, Kepler, and Gilbert; of the chemists Robert Boyle and van Helmont; and of Francis Bacon, the great exponent of the philosophy of experimentation and observation. Its medical record is equally brilliant. The previous century had effected the rebirth of the clinic and of surgery. It had brought new departures in botany and anatomy. It had seen the dawn of a scientific psychopathology, a new epidemiology, and the application of chemistry to medicine. All these branches of medicine continued to develop during the seventeenth century. In addition, two most important fields were opened up, those of physiology and microscopic anatomy. The seventeenth century sees a first peak of physiological and microscopic research. A second one will be observed around the middle of the nineteenth century. The compound microscope was invented around 1600, allowing observation beyond the range accessible to the unarmed senses. The passive observation of the previous century was supplemented by active experimentation, and anatomy developed into physiology, "animated anatomy." Function was no longer guessed at. The newly won knowledge of structure was extended to the study of function. Experiments were performed on a wider scale than ever before. Experimental pathology was practiced by a Zambeccari, Lower, Brunner, and Willis. The results of experimentation were rarely satisfactory, since this would have required a knowledge of microscopy, chemistry, or electricity not possessed by the seventeenth-century experimenter.

The greatest physiological advance of the seventeenth century, and perhaps of all times, was the discovery of the circulation of the blood. The theories of Galen concerning the movement of the blood have already been described. These theories were dominant until the seventeenth century. The first suggestion of the existence of the pulmonary circulation is found in Ibn an-Nafis (about 1210–1280) of Cairo. In the West, the first hint is given in a theological book by the unfortunate Spanish physician, Michael Servetus, who was burned as a heretic by Calvin in 1553 at the age of forty-two. Similar suggestions are put forward in the work of the Italian anatomist Columbus (died 1560), but these may have been derived from Servetus. There is no doubt, however, that Andrea Cesalpino (1524–1603), the physician to Pope Clement VIII already mentioned as a botanist, not only used the expression "circulation," but also had some rudimentary notion of the existence of the major and minor circulation.

The credit for establishing the fact of the circulation of the blood goes nevertheless to the Englishman William Harvey (1578–1657), who had studied in Padua under Fabricius ab Aquapendente. In Harvey's *De Motu Cordis*, published in 1628, the circulation of the blood was not merely put forward as a theory; it was proved by morphological, mathematical, and experimental arguments. Harvey's lecture notes show that he had entertained these ideas at least since 1616, the year of Shakespeare's death. Harvey differed from his forerunners in that his approach was not merely speculative or anatomical, but, in addition, experimental and quantitative.

Another modern aspect of his approach was the fact that he isolated his phenomenon. Harvey was concerned only with the mechanical process of circulation. He left open the question as to what else happened to the blood in the heart, liver, and brain. His argument took no account of the Galenic theory of the development of "spirits" in these organs, though he may well have believed in it himself. Harvey's approach was mechanistic in accordance with the prevailing attitude of his time. He looked upon both man and animal as machines. Fortunately he used this approach only in the particular case of circulation, which happens to be of a mechanical nature. He did not attempt to formulate any general laws of life on a purely mechanical basis, and thus he escaped the pitfalls which the iatromechanists were to encounter.

It would, however, be wrong to see in Harvey a fullfledged modern scientist. Harvey was full of "old-fashioned" philosophical ideas and arguments. It is typical of him that in the process of destroying one of Galen's main theories he was extremely anxious to quote Galen in support of his own observations. He was a child of classical antiquity, and a confirmed disciple of Aristotle, in believing the heart to be the central organ of the body and blood to be the principle of life. Like other Aristotelians, he was looking for circulatory processes everywhere. Even his Royalism may have contributed to his discovery, for he thought of the heart as the "king" of the body.

Harvey's first proof was based on morphological arguments drawn from the dissection and vivisection of animals. He pointed to the structure of the valves of the heart, the structure of the great vessels, the absence of pores in the septum, and the location of the vessels which short-circuit the lung in fetal circulation. He showed that in order to move from the right to the left side of the heart all blood had to pass through the lungs. The structure of the valves of the veins, which Harvey's teacher Fabricius had so ably described but so wrongly interpreted, supported the assumption of an exclusively centripetal movement of the blood in these vessels.

Harvey's second argument was of a mathematical and

quantitative nature. He measured the mass of blood that passed through the heart in a given time. In the case of a sheep with a total blood volume of four pounds, he estimated that the mass was 1,000 scruples, or 3½ pounds, within half an hour. He then showed that the body was unable to produce such masses in such a short time and that the blood mass could be kept constant only in a system of circulation.

Experiments with snakes showed that ligation of the vena cava left the heart empty, while ligation of the aorta accumulated blood in the heart. This confirmed Harvey's hypothesis of the one-way direction of the bloodstream. The routine bandaging in bloodletting was used for simple experiments on the same problem. Tight application of the bandage compressed the artery and stopped the pulse; looser bandaging produced stasis in the veins. A vein which was emptied between two valves by centripetal pressure did not refill from above. (Incidentally it is amazing that the age-old practice of bloodletting, which was always done below, not above, the bandage, had never produced doubts about the Galenic theory.) Harvey used additional miscellaneous arguments, such as the fact that poisons are distributed by circulation. There was one great gap in Harvey's arguments. Unfamiliar with the use of the microscope, he was unable to show how blood circulated from the arteries into the veins. This gap was to be filled through the discovery of the capillaries by Malpighi.

Harvey's interest in embryology and comparative anatomy, already apparent in his book on the motion of the heart, found its full expression in his *De Generatione Animalium* published in 1651. Here he opposed the accepted theory of preformation, which held that all organs were completely present in the germ and that growth was exclusively quantitative. In its place he favored epigenesis, the gradual building up of the embryo. His dictum, *Ex ovo omnia*, reversed the older opinion that the only active part in generation was played by the male sperm. However, he remained unaware of the true process of fecundation, the explanation of which posed a problem solvable only in the nineteenth century.

Harvey's discovery of the circulation of the blood naturally encountered violent opposition and even resulted in a falling-off of his personal practice. He seems to have been an indifferent practitioner in any case. His Royalist political views made him unpopular with many. He was court physician to Charles I and paid unswerving loyalty to his king during the great English revolution.

On the other hand acceptance of his discovery was not lacking, and almost immediately two logical conclusions were drawn from the new information: the possibility of injecting medicaments intravenously, and the possibility of transfusing blood. Intravenous injection was undertaken by Sir Christopher Wren, assisted by Boyle and Wilkins (1656), Major (1662), and Elsholtz (1665). But the practice at this stage often led to thrombosis and embolism so that it lapsed, not to be taken up again until the nineteenth century. Richard Lower transfused blood from animal to animal in 1665. Jean Denis of Paris successfully transfused animal blood to an anemic sixteen-year-old male in 1667. Later accidents in his practice led to abandonment of the technique, which was resumed only in the nineteenth century and did not become safe until the twentieth century. If Esquirol is right in claiming that the tremendous increase of bloodletting in the seventeenth century was partially due to the impact of Harvey's publication on medical thought, this can be listed as another, less desirable, consequence of Harvey's great discovery.

Circulation was not the only field of physiology to develop in the seventeenth century. Some very important observations were made concerning the physiology of respiration. The great English chemist, Robert Boyle (1627–1691), seventh son and fourteenth child of the first Earl of Cork, discovered that animal life is not dependent on air in general but rather on one particular component of the air. (This discovery is usually and erroneously credited to John Mayow,

a younger contemporary of Boyle.) Robert Hooke (1635–
1703) showed experimentally that the mechanical movement
of the thorax was not the essential element in respiration. He
demonstrated that life could be maintained in an animal,
even after removal of the thorax wall, by using bellows to
blow air through the trachea into the lungs. The difference
in color between venous and arterial blood was eventually
connected with respiration by the same Richard Lower
(1631–1691) who pioneered transfusion. He showed that this
color change took place in the lungs. It is noteworthy that
all three men were among the founders and leading spirits
of the English Royal Society.

Jean-Baptiste van Helmont (1577–1644) introduced a very
fruitful criterion into the field of digestion physiology. He
described digestion as a series of fermentations. Van Helmont was an admirer of Paracelsus and, like his master, was
simultaneously a keen chemist and a mystic philosopher.
His interest in theological problems was as intense as that of
Boyle or Newton. He identified hydrochloric acid in the
stomach. He is remembered for many other scientific accomplishments, including the discovery of carbon dioxide ("spirit
of wood"), the invention of the term "gas," and the elimination of the age-old belief that mucus in head colds is secreted
by the brain. Another early pioneer of digestion physiology
was Regner de Graaf (1641–1673), a pupil of the iatrochemist
Sylvius and a friend of Leeuwenhoek. He experimented on
the pancreas and gall bladder of dogs.

The physiology of digestion and respiration could not yet
make the same advances as the physiology of circulation since
the underlying problems were chemical, and chemistry had
not yet developed to the extent that physics had. The same
handicap, insufficient development of the basic sciences, also
limited the otherwise remarkable work of Sanctorius of
Padua (1561–1636) on "insensible perspiration," that is, metabolism. Sanctorius was one of the pioneers of modern
physiology. His quantitative approach to physiological problems led him to invent new instruments, such as clinical ther-

mometers and a pulse clock. The decerebration experiments of Johann Bohn, Boyle, Redi, Perrault, and Swammerdam initiated a revived study of the physiology of the nervous system. Muscle physiology was cultivated by Steno, Borelli, Willis, Glisson, and others.

Through his discovery (1661) of the capillaries, Marcello Malpighi (1628–1694) completed the work of Harvey on the circulation of the blood. Malpighi's pioneer microscopic work was by no means limited to this discovery. He made the first microscopic analysis of the structures of the lung, the spleen, the kidney, the liver, and the skin. He described sensory papillae and taste buds. Malpighi's name has deservedly become an eponym for a number of structures. In addition to being a microscopist, he was an outstanding embryologist, plant anatomist, and zoologist. In short, he was one of the great scientists of the times.

The rise of microscopy is usually connected with the name of Anton van Leeuwenhoek (1632–1723), a draper and amateur scientist from Delft, Holland. Many of Leeuwenhoek's numerous discoveries with the microscope are of medical importance. For instance, his were the first descriptions of bacteria, of the striped muscle, and of the spermatozoon. Other early microscopists were Francisco Redi (1626–1697), who dealt the first blow to the theory of spontaneous generation; the Jesuit Athanasius Kirchner (1602–1680), who explained infectious disease by the presence of microscopical worms in the blood (the "worms" he saw under his low-power microscope were probably red blood corpuscles); Robert Hooke, mentioned earlier for his physiological work, who gave the name "cell" to formations he observed in plants; and Jan Swammerdam (1637–1680), who first described the red corpuscles.

The most important event in gross anatomy during the seventeenth century was probably the discovery of the lymphatic system, the nature of which was gradually unveiled by Aselli (1622), Pecquet (1651), Bartholinus (1652), and Rudbeck (1653). The names of seventeenth-century anato-

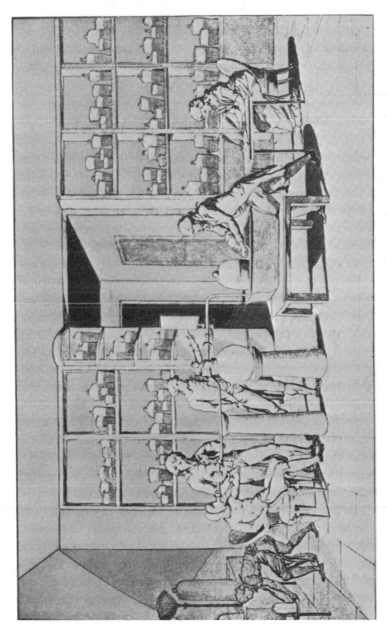

FIGURE 11. Lavoisier experimenting on respiration (drawing by Mme. Lavoisier).

mists still used as eponyms in gross anatomy include those of Wirsung, Bartholinus, Cowper, Meibom, Brunner, Peyer, Stensen, and de Graaf. The fact that the structures to which these names are attached belong mainly to the realm of the ducts and glands (Wirsung's duct, Brunner's glands, Graafian follicles) shows that these organs were the center of interest for seventeenth-century anatomists. The interest in glands was perhaps a result of the iatrochemical trends of the time. Comparative anatomy had been rediscovered in the preceding century by Belon, Rondelet, and Coiter. Their work was continued in the seventeenth century by Edward Tyson (1655–1708), who studied the chimpanzee, and the Parisian group centering round the scientist-architect Claude Perrault (1613–1688). Perrault died from an infected wound which he acquired while dissecting a camel.

It was a great temptation to apply the fragmentary results of the two budding new basic sciences, physics and chemistry, to clinical medicine. This attempt took the form of two powerful movements, iatromathematics (or iatrophysics) and iatrochemistry. With iatrophysics a pathology of solids returned to the foreground after fourteen hundred years during which humoral pathology had reigned supreme. Iatrophysics flourished chiefly in the south of Europe, while iatrochemistry was more popular in the northern latitudes. An outstanding iatrophysicist was the French physician-philosopher René Descartes (1596–1650). To Descartes man was a machine except for the pineal gland, where the rational soul was located. The dualism of Descartes facilitated physiological research, but created problems that still plague us. The center of iatrophysics was, of course, Italy, where Galileo Galilei (1564–1642) of Padua created a new quantitative, mathematical, and experimental form of physics (the law of fall) and, through his telescopic discoveries, brought about the victory of the heliocentric system of Nicholas Copernicus (1473–1558), a system that undermined all the ancient authorities. Giovanni Borelli (1608–1679) was successful in analyzing the action of muscles along mechanical lines. But application of the same principle by him and Giorgio Baglivi (1668–1706) to the function of glands, and to the phenomena of respiration and digestion, produced rather absurd results. The close connection between physics and medicine was profitable for ophthalmology. Physicists like Descartes, Mariotte, and Scheiner made many contributions to physiological optics.

The iatrochemists were never accepted to the extent that the iatromechanists were. This was probably due to the undeveloped state of chemistry. The outstanding iatrochemist was François de la Boë (1614–1672), also known as Sylvius of Leyden and not to be confused with the sixteenth-century Parisian anatomist, Sylvius. This Sylvius tried to classify diseases according to "acidosis" or "alkalosis." If to Borelli renal function, for example, was a purely mechanical problem, it was purely chemical to Sylvius. Thomas Willis (1621–1675) interpreted fevers as fermentations before Sylvius.

As a whole both movements, iatrophysics and iatrochemistry, were bound to be failures. Their history is interesting nevertheless as demonstrating the danger of premature application of basic scientific data to clinical medicine. It also makes clear the tremendous amount of basic data, so-called "useless knowledge," that is necessary in order to make such applications fruitful. Further, it illustrates the urgent need always felt by scientists for a basic theory which will bring order to the chaos of raw data. A reaction followed, in which the proponents of "vitalism" claimed that life phenomena could not be explained in terms of mere physics or chemistry. One of the first manifestations of this reaction was Glisson's theory of irritability as a special quality of animal tissues.

Iatrochemical and iatrophysical theories could make little contribution to the advance of clinical medicine. Advances in clinical medicine in the seventeenth century had to be made independently of these theories. Nevertheless this century was one of great achievements in the clinical field, a fact which is all too often overshadowed by the purely scien-

tific advances of the period. Even laymen like La Roche-
foucauld, Saint-Simon, and La Bruyère show an acuteness
and a detachment in observing humans that has something
"clinical" in it. It is somewhat unjust to make Thomas
Sydenham (1624–1689), the "English Hippocrates," the only
representative of this clinical achievement and to look upon
him as the only practical man of his time, free from the
sterile theorizing of his contemporaries. Without intending
to minimize his true merits, it must be stated that Sydenham
was not free from harboring theories himself, theories often
just as inadequate as those of his contemporaries. Nor were
many of the outstanding iatromechanists and iatrochemists
inferior to Sydenham when it came to clinical observation
and description.

Sydenham, originally a captain in Cromwell's army, came
into medicine relatively late. He received his medical license
at the age of thirty-nine. A friend of Boyle and the philoso-
pher-physician John Locke, he acquired their direct approach, putting observation above everything. In this respect
the parallel between Sydenham and Hippocrates is undoubtedly justified. He was also a Hippocratist in maintaining the theory of "coction." On the other hand, his plan to
observe and classify disease according to species as if they
were plants—a plan which he did not carry out, thereby avoiding the opprobrium that befell those who were unfortunate
enough to do so in the following century—is as far from
Hippocrates as it could be. For better or worse Hippocrates
observed sick people, not diseases. Symptoms served him as
indicators of the status of the patient, not as a basis of classification.

Since the diseases most prevalent in Sydenham's time
were the epidemic diseases, the "fevers," it is not surprising
that one of his main theories dealt with the genesis of epidemic diseases. This was the theory of the "epidemic constitution," a revival and extension of a Hippocratic idea.
Though modern doctors must humbly recognize that they are
still very deficient in explaining the phenomena of epidemics,

it can be said that this theory in its vagueness did little either to explain the data or to further the development of epidemiology.

Sydenham's greatness lies in his clinical observation and his relatively reasonable treatment. He is justly famous for his studies of malarial fevers, dysentery, measles, scarlet fever, and the chorea minor which bears his name. His best-known work is his treatise on gout, of which he was a sufferer. His treatise on hysteria, in which he claimed that half of his nonfever patients, male and female, suffered from what is called today "psychosomatic" disease, is a masterpiece of sober description.

In his attempt to support the *vis medicatrix naturae* (the self-healing tendencies of the body), Sydenham based his treatment primarily on experience, not theory. His methods differed considerably from those of most of his contemporaries, although even he did not escape altogether the temptations to extensive bloodletting. He wanted to complement a strict classification of disease with a strict *methodus medendi* (method of treatment). His individualization of diseases made him sympathetic to the idea of specific remedies. It is much to his credit that he, a Puritan, adopted, after initial resistance, the one great specific that appeared at this time—quinine, "the Jesuit powder," imported from Peru in the 1630's. That a former cavalry officer should regard horseback riding as a panacea, equally effective in consumption and hysteria, is not surprising.

The effects of the impact of quinine on medicine were many and various, quite apart from the fact that it cured the most frequent disease of the period. It made possible the objective separation of malaria from other fevers. It seemed to confirm the ideas of specific diseases and specific remedies. Above all, quinine cured without producing any of the "evacuations" claimed necessary by the Galenists and humoral pathologists. This fact undermined to a considerable extent the traditional pharmacological and pathological theories.

Among the great clinicians of the century can be numbered most of the men who were, from the modern viewpoint, such failures as medical theoreticians. The iatrophysicist Baglivi, for example, once he entered the sick room, made it a principle to abandon all his theories and to act in a truly Hippocratic fashion. He made valuable contributions to the pathology of typhoid, which he called mesenteric fever. The iatrochemist Thomas Willis, who was just as sturdy a Royalist as Sydenham was a Cromwellian, is now mainly remembered for his accomplishments in brain anatomy (the circle of Willis). He first described the two antagonistic elements of the vegetative nervous system; he recognized the role of the brain cortex; he experimented on brain localizations; he coined the terms psychology, neurology, and comparative anatomy; and he found the reflex and named it. Yet Willis also discovered the sweetness of diabetic urine and gave excellent descriptions of puerperal fever, typhoid fever, myasthenia gravis, and hysteria. Willis was one of the very first to regard hysteria as a disease of the nervous system. He gave one of the earliest descriptions of general paresis. Francis Glisson's (1597–1677) description of rickets is so excellent that it has overshadowed an earlier description of the same disease by Reusner in 1582. Glisson is also known as an anatomist. Richard Morton (1635–1698) left two great books on pulmonary tuberculosis and malaria. He was the first to conceive the idea of differentiating malarial fevers from other fevers through the exclusive therapeutic effect of quinine on the former.

Many of the clinical accomplishments of the seventeenth century were based on the increasing integration of pathological anatomical data with clinical observation. This holds true of the fine description of tuberculosis by Sylvius, who revived bedside teaching at Leyden. By means of autopsies Johann Jacob Wepfer (1620–1695), the head of the Schaffhouse school and pioneer of experimental toxicology, was able to show that brain hemorrhage caused the mysterious "strokes" and apoplexies. Raymond Vieussens (1641–1717) of Montpellier gave excellent clinical and pathological ana-tomical descriptions of the two main valvular diseases, aortic insufficiency (widening of the aortic valve), and mitral stenosis (narrowing of the mitral valve). Vieussens also con-tributed much to the anatomy of the nervous system. Giovanni Maria Lancisi (1654–1720), the body physician of three popes, was equally masterly in his description of heart diseases and as a malariologist. Lancisi probably came closer than any one of his predecessors, certainly than all his followers up to the middle of the nineteenth century, to an understanding of the connection between the mosquito and malaria. His practical sanitation work was admirable. All existing pathological anatomical knowledge was compiled by Théophile Bonet of Geneva (1620–1689) in his famous *Sepulchretum.*

Many of the seventeenth-century clinicians opened up entirely new fields. Bernardino Ramazzini (1633–1714) con-tributed his classic on occupational diseases. Tropical dis-eases were studied to a large extent by Dutch clinicians. Bontius and Tulpius—the Dr. Tulp of the famous Rembrandt painting—gave the first descriptions of beriberi. Willem Piso (1563–1636) learned from the Brazilian Indians the use of ipecacuanha in amebic dysentery (its alkaloid, emetine, is still used for the same purpose). Mention should be made of the well-illustrated work of Marco Aurelio Severino (1580–1656) on surgical pathology, especially tumors. Surgery maintained the level attained in the sixteenth century in the work of such men as Fabricius of Hilden in Bern and Richard Wiseman in England, but it made no noticeable progress.

In the seventeenth century obstetrics, which for several millennia had been the domain of midwives, became more and more part of the domain of the male doctor. As surgeons were less analphabetic than midwives, this led to an increas-ingly scientific development of the obstetrical art. The fact that kings used "male midwives" for their queens and mistresses facilitated the acceptance of obstetricians by a reluctant public. Outstanding in the seventeenth century were the Dutch obstetricians led by Hendrik van Deventer (1651–1724) and the French group led by François Mauriceau (1637–1709). Mauriceau described tubal pregnancy and did away with such errors as the separation of the pelvic bones during delivery. In spite of these advances in obstetrics, the seventeenth century still saw great midwives like M. L. Bourgeois (1564–1644) and Justine Siegemundin (1650–1705).

The seventeenth century also saw the birth of a systematic and scientific legal medicine in the great treatises of the papal physician Paolo Zacchias (1584–1659) and Johann Bohn of Leipzig (1640–1719). Jan Swammerdam discovered that the lung of the stillborn child would not swim (docimasia), a discovery first put to practical use by Johann Schreyer in 1681. Medical statistics appeared on the scene with John Grant's *Natural and Political Observations upon the Bills of Mortality*, published in 1662. Grant's work was followed by that of Sir William Petty (1623–1687), of the astronomer Edmund Halley (1656–1742), and the Prussian army chaplain J. P. Suessmilch. An early attempt to organize preventive medicine was the collegium sanitatis in Prussia (1685).

Though there were great clinicians in the seventeenth century, the average product of universities tended to exhibit sterile learning more than clinical skill and to indulge in a harmful routine of abundant purging and bloodletting in therapeutics. This type of doctor has been depicted in Molière's great satires. Molière happened to be familiar with probably the most conservative and sterile medical school of his time, the Paris faculty, the attitude of which is adequately reflected in the gossiping letters of its vampiric dean, Guy Patin. Universities in general remained medieval and were not attuned to the scientific progress of the time. Practically all the great discoveries of the century were sponsored, not by universities, but by the so-called academies and learned societies. The works of Boyle, Malpighi, and Leeuwenhoek, for example, were published in the transactions of the Royal

Society of London, which was chartered in 1662 and was an outgrowth of the "invisible college" founded in 1645. Similar free academies and scientific societies sprang up in all important European countries. The Academia del Lincei was founded in Rome in 1603, the French Academy of Science in Paris in 1665, and the Leopoldine Academy in Germany in 1677. They were the actual centers of scientific discovery and discussion up to the nineteenth century, when the universities were reformed. The seventeenth century also saw the first appearance of medical journals.

The brilliant accomplishments of the century, and the first signs of therapeutic skepticism (Daniel Ludwig, 1625–1680), should not obscure the fact that, in addition to official polypragmasy and polypharmacy, superstition was widespread and rampant, and quackery was extremely successful. This was the age of the sympathetic powder of Sir Kenelm Digby, which was supposed to heal a wound when put on the weapon which had caused it; of the "magnetic" cures of Valentine Greatrake; of the astrological medicine of Culpeper; and of the mass healing of scrofulosis (also called King's Evil) by the touch of the French and English kings. The Rosicrucian and other mystic movements flourished.

Italy was still the leader of Europe in medicine and science, in spite of its political decline. France was stagnant, but Holland and England had become great powers in science and medicine as well as in politics and art. Germany had passed through one of the worst periods of its history, the Thirty Years' War, and was correspondingly unproductive, while little Switzerland produced an unusual number of outstanding medical men.

Chapter 11

MEDICINE IN THE EIGHTEENTH CENTURY

The remarkable achievements which characterize eighteenth-century medicine and science were realized almost without exception in the second half of that period. Only then did the great philosophical movement of the Enlightenment bear fruit in the new discoveries of medical science. For the earlier part of this century separation from the seventeenth century is largely artificial. The preoccupations of the previous century survived into its successor, often on a lower level.

Attempts to systematize medicine around simple fundamental principles continued. The success of Newton in finding basic physical laws encouraged such attempts. Much intelligence was wasted on these sterile endeavors. Iatrochemists and iatrophysicists went on with their speculations. The vitalist reaction against iatrochemistry and iatrophysics, already noted in the seventeenth century, gained momentum and reached its peak with the "animism" of Georg Ernst Stahl (1660–1734) of Halle, Germany. Stahl explained life and disease by the action of a "sensitive soul," or *anima*, which inhabited every part of the organism and prevented its spontaneous putrefaction. Stahl kept his medicine separate from his chemistry, in spite of the fact that he was one of the great chemists of his age. His phlogiston theory, which interpreted combustion as the escape of a special substance called phlogiston, was dominant up to the time of Lavoisier. Stahl's animist theory helped him gain an insight into psychopathology and psychotherapy, an insight to which his own personality—he supposedly died in a state of depression—perhaps contributed. His vitalism was carried on primarily by de Bordeu and Barthez of the Montpellier School.

Stahl was one of the luminaries of the newly founded University of Halle (1694), the home both of Pietism, a new mystic variety of Protestantism, and of the enlightened philosophies of Christian Wolff and Christian Thomasius, a famous opponent of witch-hunting. Stahl himself was a Pietist. He never achieved the popularity of his colleague and rival, Friedrich Hoffmann (1660–1742), inventor of a mechanist system but also an able practitioner whose slogan was "Reasoning plus experience." Hoffmann regarded the body as a kind of hydraulic machine, kept going by a hypothetical fluid circulating in the nervous system. Notable among his many clinical descriptions are those of rubella (called "German" measles as a consequence of his description), chlorosis, and the diseases of the pancreas and liver. He made a praiseworthy attempt to reduce the particularly luxuriant pharmacopoeia of the time to ten or twelve effective remedies.

William Cullen of Edinburgh (1712–1790) founded a medical system on the assumption that the basic phenomenon of life and disease was a "nervous force." His pupil, the alcoholic John Brown (1735–1788), derived from this another system that was actually a revival of ancient methodism, which received favorably in Germany, Italy, and the United States. Every disease was to Brown either *sthenia*, a result of overstimulation, or *asthenia*, inability to respond to stimulation. Therapeutics were correspondingly reduced to the use of stimulating and depressing agents, especially opium and alcohol.

Sydenham's suggestion for the classification of diseases in the manner of plants was taken up by the great Swedish botanist, Carl von Linné (1707–1778), already the author of the best basic system of classification for the animal and plant kingdoms. The classificatory systems for disease developed by Linné and others were practically without value, since diseases are neither plants nor animals, and medicine is not a science like botany and zoology. While the older medicine had suffered from a lack of disease entities and had been content with such over-all categories as "fevers" and "plagues," the classifiers multiplied artificial disease units to the point of absurdity. Boissier de Sauvages, for example, described twenty-four hundred diseases. Medicine has lost interest in systematics to the same extent that she has acquired actual knowledge.

The most successful clinician and medical teacher of the century was the Dutchman Hermann Boerhaave (1668–1738) of Leyden. He made Leyden, already outstanding at the time of Sylvius, the medical center of the world. Boerhaave's convincing personality and eclectic approach attracted wide attention. As an eclectic, he did not subscribe to any single system; he tried to combine features of the mechanistic, the chemical, and the direct clinical approach. Boerhaave continued bedside teaching, and his influence was felt primarily through the great number of outstanding pupils he trained.

Two great new centers of clinical medicine in the eighteenth century, Edinburgh and Vienna, were both founded by pupils of Boerhaave. The fame of Edinburgh depended on such Boerhaave pupils as the elder Alexander Monro (1697–1767) and Robert Whytt (1714–1766). Edinburgh attracted the best graduate students from the young North American colonies. Edinburgh was the only modern university in Great Britain, and therefore was also the only one to admit "dissenters," i.e., non-members of the High Church. British dissenters, like other minorities (German Jews, French Protestants), were to play an important role in the evolution of modern medicine, especially in the nineteenth century. The Vienna school was established by the Boerhaave pupils Gerard van Swieten (1700–1772) and Anton de Haen (1704–1776). The new clinical system imported into Austria by these Dutchmen quickly took root. The school soon included such outstanding practitioners as Stoerck in pharmacology, Stoll in epidemiology, and von Plenck in dermatology. Its early decline has been attributed to bureaucratic pressures. Boerhaave's pupils were also influential in Russia and Prussia.

In spite of the preoccupation with systems, the study of individual diseases and the isolation of new disease entities made continued progress in the eighteenth century. Great Britain remained outstanding in the practical fields in which it had excelled in the previous century. Quakers, especially, produced a number of outstanding doctors in the eighteenth and nineteenth centuries, since medicine was the only learned profession open to dissenters in England at that time. The Edinburgh-trained Quaker John Fothergill (1712–1780) is remembered for his studies of diphtheria and neuralgia. Another Quaker, John C. Lettsom (1744–1815), paid special attention to alcoholism.

Yet another outstanding English physician of the period was John Huxham (1692–1768), a pupil of Boerhaave. He studied fevers, primarily the "putrid malignant" and "slow nervous" varieties—the contemporary names for typhus and typhoid. Another Boerhaave pupil, Robert Whytt of Edinburgh, made a great number of valuable neurological observations on reflex and shock. He still called reflex "sympathy." He was the first to describe tuberculous meningitis in children. George Cheyne (1671–1743) dealt with obesity, with which he himself was afflicted, and neurotic behavior, which he called "the English disease." William Withering (1741–1799) of Birmingham, a clinician, botanist, and social reformer, introduced digitalis into orthodox medicine after learning of the use of foxglove for dropsy from an old woman in 1775. The assimilation of folk remedies (see also Fowler, Jenner, and so forth) was a specialty of Enlightenment doctors. One of the keenest clinicians of the age was William Heberden (1710–1801), from whom come the first classic descriptions of angina pectoris (1768), of varicella (chickenpox) (1767), and of nodules formed in the fingers in arthritis deformans. Heberden's *Essay on Mithridatum and Theriaca* (1745) made a contribution to the revision of the pharmacopoeia, undertaken at this time and directed against magic and ineffectual remedies.

The practical trend of the eighteenth century was by no means limited to Great Britain. The Spaniard Gaspar Casal (1691–1759) described pellagra for the first time in 1735. Théodore Tronchin (1709–1781) of Geneva, a favorite pupil of Boerhaave and a promoter of inoculation, became, through sensible simplification of treatments, the most popular practitioner of the eighteenth century. Germany recovered from the shock of the Thirty Years' War and contributed, besides Hoffmann, such able clinicians as Paul Werlhof (1699–1767), an outstanding student of exanthemata, and Christian Selle (1748–1800). The tubercular nature of Pott's disease was first stated by Johann Platner of Chemnitz in 1744.

The eighteenth century witnessed the full social emancipation of surgery and the consequent rapid growth of this discipline, especially in France. The gratitude of King Louis XIV, who was cured of his anal fistula in 1686 by the royal surgeon Felix, opened the way to the rehabilitation of the surgical profession in France. The absolute monarchs and their ministers began some bookkeeping and realized therewith that better medical care for soldiers and peasants would pay. This better care could only be realized through the mass of surgeons, not through a very few learned physicians. This was given a practical basis by the foundation of the Royal Academy of Surgery in 1731 by Mareschal, who succeeded Felix as the royal surgeon, and La Peyronie. Among the many outstanding French surgeons of this century mention should be made of Pierre Dionis (died 1718), who laid the foundations of surgical anatomy; Jean Louis Petit (1674–1750), who performed the first mastoid operation, wrote an outstanding book on bone pathology, and recommended removal of metastatic lymph glands in cancer; and Pierre-Joseph Desault (1744–1795), a teacher of Bichat and prominent both as a surgical anatomist and as a pathological anatomist. The fame of French surgeons in the field of pathological anatomy has somewhat obscured the accomplishments of the French physicians of this period. However, the work of Senac in the field of heart diseases and of Portal in the description of phthisis is noteworthy.

The British, too, produced outstanding surgeons, the greatest of whom was John Hunter (1728–1793). A Scotsman, like so many outstanding British medical men of the century, Hunter was the key figure in the transformation of surgery from a mere craft into an experimental science. Not that he was alone in this movement. Earlier the French surgeons F. Pourfour du Petit (1664–1741) and Nicolas Saucerotte (1741–1814) had used animal experiments to illuminate problems in neurosurgery and neuro-anatomy. Hunter's most important single contribution was his experimental work on inflammation. However, his claim to fame lies not so much in any individual accomplishment as in his pioneer activities in many fields. Not only did he open up an era of brilliant accomplishments in pathological anatomy in Great Britain, he also contributed greatly to the knowledge of comparative anatomy. He trained many able pupils. He initiated scientific dentistry in Great Britain, a new field which had been largely delineated by Pierre Fauchard in his treatise *Le Chirurgien Dentiste,* published in 1728. Other prominent English surgeons of the time were William Cheselden, Charles White, and Percival Pott.

The foundation of institutions for the teaching of obstetrics marks the continuing advance of this discipline during the eighteenth century. The first such institution was founded in Paris in 1720. Obstetrics continued to flourish in France under de la Motte and Jean Louis Baudelocque, and in other Continental countries it was fostered by such men as Palfyn, Camper, and K. K. Siebold. Obstetrics came into its own in England under the leadership of two Scotsmen, William Smellie (1697–1763) and William Hunter (1718–1783), the older brother of John Hunter.

In 1761 Giovanni Battista Morgagni of Padua published, at the age of seventy-nine, his monumental book, *On the Sites and Causes of Disease.* In this great work the pathological anatomical trend of the century came to a climax. Morgagni's treatise on pathological anatomy, based on about seven hundred dissections by the author and his teacher Valsalva, was superior to all its forerunners in its systematic character, its thoroughness, and the particularly successful correlation of clinical symptoms and autopsy findings. The book held to the old-fashioned "head-to-feet" arrangement of Egyptian times, and the author—still a humoralist in many ways—was hardly conscious of the full consequences of his work. But it opened a new era in the practice of medicine and surgery. Emphasis on the explanation of disease now definitely shifted from concentration on general conditions and humors to the study of localized change in organs; and the changes were causally connected with clinical symptoms. The Scot Matthew Baillie (1761–1823), pupil and nephew of the Hunters, made use of the new approach in his valuable textbook on pathological anatomy (1793). It also finds expression in the work of Eduard Sandifort (1740–1819) of Leyden.

In the same year that Morgagni's *magnum opus* appeared, Leopold Auenbrugger (1722–1809) of Vienna published his *Inventum Novum,* a landmark in the field of physical diagnosis. Little noticed during its author's lifetime, this work is now regarded as the most noteworthy contribution to medicine of the old Vienna school. In this short treatise Auenbrugger taught his new technique of examining the chest by percussion and demonstrated the services that the new technique could render in the diagnosis and prognosis of chest diseases. One has always assumed that Auenbrugger, a gifted amateur, musician, composer of several operas, and the son of an innkeeper, had learned percussion through handling barrels in his father's cellar. Erna Lesky has discovered the more essential fact that van Swieten, Auenbrugger's teacher, applied percussion to the abdomen with ascites. In spite of the humoral ideas of its author, Auenbrugger's work expresses the same trend toward localization that is present in Morgagni's pathological anatomy. It also reflects the increasing desire for more exact methods of physical diagnosis. Clinical thermometry became more and more popular during the eighteenth century. Outstanding protagonists of temperature-taking were de Haen and the Scots, Martin and Curry. As early as 1707 Sir John Floyer had recommended timing the pulse with appropriate watches.

In medical science the outstanding figure of the eighteenth century was Albrecht von Haller (1708–1777), a Swiss pupil of Boerhaave. At the age of twenty-eight Haller became professor in the newly founded University of Goettingen, where he created an active center of scientific research. Haller, who included botany and poetry among his many interests, did valuable work in anatomy, especially the anatomy of vessels. But his most important contribution lay in the field of experimental physiology. He replaced mechanical or chemical-physiological speculations with a step-by-step inquiry into the actual physiology of various organs. His experimental demonstration of the difference between the primary quality of the muscle ("irritability") and the primary quality of the nerve ("sensibility") had a wide and long-lasting influence upon medical thought. While the importance of the experiment lay in the fact that Haller had distinguished between nerve impulses and muscular contraction, an unfortunate consequence was the subsequent misuse of the data. The notion of irritability, especially, was abused in medical circles. Haller was a great encyclopedist, and his eight-volume *Elementa Physiologiae* contains all that was known of physiology up to his time. The physiologist Magendie used to say angrily that whenever a man thought he had performed a new experiment, he always found it already described in Haller. The latter's Enlightenment philosophy appears clearest in his political novels.

The English clergyman, Stephen Hales (1677–1761), made valuable contributions to hemodynamics by developing techniques for measuring blood pressure, the capacity of the heart, and the velocity of the blood current. William Hewson

(1749–1774), a pupil of the Hunters, did his most important experimental work on the coagulation of the blood.

This was the century in which chemistry came of age, and those fields of physiology which offered primarily chemical problems were now able to progress considerably. The experiments of the naturalists René Antoine de Réaumur (1683–1757) and Lazaro Spallanzani (1729–1799) showed clearly that digestion was neither a purely mechanical process nor a process of putrification. They demonstrated that it depended rather on chemical solution. Spallanzani, one of the most remarkable scientists of all times, made valuable experiments to disprove spontaneous generation. He also practiced artificial insemination in animals and demonstrated the phenomenon of tissue respiration.

In 1757 carbon dioxide was rediscovered by Joseph Black of Glasgow. In 1766 Cavendish discovered hydrogen, and six years later Rutherford discovered nitrogen. Oxygen was discovered by Scheele in 1772 and by Priestley in 1774, although its true nature was realized only by Lavoisier in 1775. This new knowledge of the gases composing the air eventually made possible identification of that "unknown part" of the air, originally posited by Boyle, which was essential for respiration. At the same time it brought about an understanding of the process of combustion, chemically identical to respiration. The unveiling of the mystery of respiration, the decisive scientific contribution of the eighteenth century to medicine, was the work of Antoine Laurent Lavoisier (1743–1794). It is impossible to deal here with the many aspects of the work of a man who laid the foundations of modern quantitative chemistry as a whole and created the greater part of modern chemical terminology. It is equally impossible to go into the details of Lavoisier's personal life, although it should at least be mentioned that he was executed by the revolutionary government in 1794, not by reason of his scientific activities, but because he had been a member of the hated tax bureaucracy of the *ancien régime*.

In his memoir of 1777 on oxidation and respiration Lavoisier stated that respiration essentially consisted of an intake of oxygen and a corresponding elimination of carbon dioxide, a fact expressed today by the respiratory quotient. In 1780, together with the astronomer Laplace, he showed that in respiration the same amount of oxygen is used, and the same amount of heat is produced, as in the burning of coal—a fact basic to modern calorimetry. In 1789 he worked with Seguin to measure the changing oxygen intake during work, eating, and rest. Lavoisier's work was extended by the mathematician Lagrange, who found in 1791 that the chemical changes during respiration do not take place in the lung, and by Spallanzani, who in 1803 localized the changes in the tissues. A fitting epitome of Lavoisier's life is the remark of Lagrange after Lavoisier's execution: "It took but an instant to chop off his head, yet a hundred years will not suffice to produce one like it."

Modern work in embryology started in this period with Caspar Friedrich Wolff (1733–1794). Wolff's results influenced the dispute between preformationists and epigenesists in favor of the latter. Wolff was the only outstanding microscopist of the century. Apart from him, microscopical work came to a perplexing standstill. Gross anatomy made no essential progress except in the field of surgical anatomy. The discovery of Luigi Galvani (1737-1798) and Alessandro Volta (1745–1827) that electrical processes are involved in the function of muscles and nerves was to bear rich fruit in the following century. Its immediate result was the appearance of therapeutic fads and fakes.

In spite of respectable clinical work and great scientific progress, the most characteristic medical advances of the eighteenth century are those most directly associated with the philosophy of the Enlightenment. This philosophy, born in seventeenth-century England, culminated in the work of such great Frenchmen as Diderot, d'Alembert, la Mettrie, Voltaire, and Rousseau. Well represented in America by Franklin and Jefferson, this philosophy underlay the American Revolution as well as the French. It shifted the center of interest from preoccupation with the fate of the soul in another world toward improvement of conditions in this

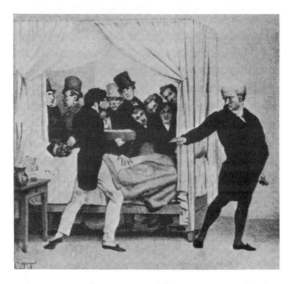

FIGURE 12. Caricature of Broussais ("Ninety more leeches . . . and continue a strict diet").

world. Such changes were thought to be possible through "enlightenment," a rational approach to all problems, combined with the dissemination of knowledge to the largest possible extent. The applied aspects of science were emphasized. It is no accident that the term "social science" appeared first in the writings of the Enlightenment. Climate, which since Hippocrates had explained everything, became now less important than social conditions, which changed very drastically in the so-called Industrial Revolution. One can influence social conditions, while climate is inaccessible!

The rapid spread of this new philosophy led to the disappearance of belief in the devil and "possession." Thus mental disease again became a legitimate preoccupation of the doctor. Recognition that mental disorder was a disease, rather than a kind of possession, sin, crime, or vice, also made possible a more humane treatment of the insane, who up to this time had been kept under atrocious conditions, often in chains. The new therapeutic optimism was sometimes

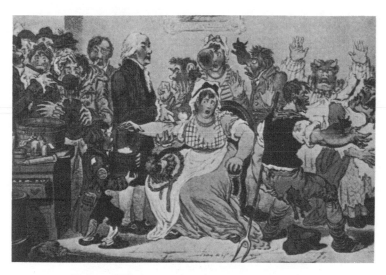

FIGURE 13. Caricature of cowpox vaccination.

implemented by such cruel mechanical means as Erasmus Darwin's rotating chair, but it led nonetheless to a new understanding of psychotherapy on the part of men like Haslam, Scheidemantel, and Tissot. Social pressures were now considered as causative factors in mental disease. The new scientific and humane approach to psychiatry is typically represented by Philippe Pinel (1755–1826), who wrote a medicophilosophical treatise on mental alienation. He removed the chains from his insane patients in the Bicêtre hospital of Paris in 1794. Aiding Pinel in his advancement of psychiatry was his reputation in other fields. He was a highly esteemed nosographer, a member of the influential philosophical school of the *Idéologues,* and an outstanding clinician. His work was quickly taken up and developed by a very brilliant school of French psychiatrists. The new psychiatry was represented in England by men like William Battie, Thomas Arnold, and William Perfect; in Germany by J. C. Reil, a prominent freemason; and in the United States by Benjamin Rush. Hypochondria was the fashionable

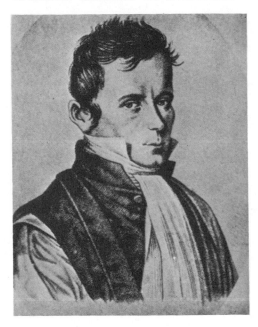

FIGURE 14. René Théophile Hyacinthe Laennec.

psychological disease of the century. Esther Fischer-Homberger has followed the checkered career of the disease (which is still with us as "neurosis") under the labels of melancholy, spinal irritation, neurasthenia, and hysteria.

The new approach of the Enlightenment stimulated that field of medicine now called public health. In all branches of medicine the preventive idea came now to the fore-ground. People no longer felt indifferent toward the atrocious health conditions in armies, navies, prisons, and hospitals. The sanitary reform of prisons—overrun by typhus, typhoid fever, and tuberculosis—was primarily the work of the English philanthropist John Howard (1726–1790). The great Lavoisier himself studied the problems of hygienic prison buildings and appropriate sewers. Improvement in military medicine was brought about by Sir John Pringle (1707–1782), a Scottish pupil of Boerhaave and surgeon general of the British armies from 1742 to 1758 and by the Goettingen professor E. G. Baldinger (1738–1804). The Scotsmen James Lind (1716–1794) and Thomas Trotter (1760–1832) led a valiant and effective fight against scurvy, typhus, and other diseases which were killing large numbers of sailors in the navy. Lind proved experimentally the preventive and curative value of citrus fruits in scurvy. He baked the clothes of newly recruited sailors, who were often just released from the pestilent, louse-ridden prisons of the times, and thus checked the spread of typhus in the British navy. He also invented a method of distilling sea water.

Improvements in hospital conditions were made during this period, particularly after J. R. Tenon exposed the scandalous conditions in Paris hospitals in 1788. As a result of the urgings of John Haygarth (1740–1827) of Chester, special fever wards were created for the first time in 1783. The whole field of public health was surveyed in the basic and monumental work of Johann Peter Frank (1745–1821), which was based on his extraordinarily rich experiences as a practitioner in Bitch, Baden-Baden, and Rastatt; as a professor of medicine in Goettingen, Pavia, Vienna, and Vilna; and as court physician in Bruchsal and St. Petersburg. His six-volume *Complete System of Medical Policy* was published between 1777 and 1817. This amazing book even includes elements of modern fields, such as the medicine of catastrophes and the medicine of the diseases of the wealthy. He regarded misery as the "mother of disease" and thought relief would come through the "enlightened despotism" of such philanthropic monarchs as his master, Emperor Joseph II of Austria. Frank was also a prominent clinician. He influenced and, in turn, was strongly influenced by the Lausanne hygienist S. Tissot (1728–1797).

Individual hygiene received an equal stimulus from the Enlightenment. The anatomist Peter Camper fought deformation of the foot caused by unhygienic foot gear, and another anatomist, Samuel Soemmering, led a valiant fight against the corset. The American Loyalist, Benjamin Thompson (1753–1814), who ended his career as Count Rumford and a great physicist in Munich, made remarkable studies of heating, ventilation, clothing, and food.

The most important factor in improving the health conditions of infants and children was probably the influence of the Geneva-born novelist and philosopher, Jean Jacques Rousseau. Thanks to him swaddling was discarded, and mothers returned to nursing their own babies. Rousseau's activities epitomize the effective participation of laymen in this and later public health movements. Of course, physicians like B. Faust or Rosen von Rosenstein also played a great role in this movement. The first orthopedic institute for crippled children was opened in Switzerland by Jean André Venel in 1780. The increased interest in child welfare and child health found its statistical expression in a decrease in the appalling death rate of infants and children. The medical men who were guided by the philosophy of the Enlightenment were concerned not only about children, but also about mothers, old people, deafmutes, the blind, and so forth.

One of the great contributions to the new public health movement was the general introduction of an effective preventive measure against smallpox toward the end of the century. Smallpox was one of the main causes of childhood death in this period. It is significant that it was only during the eighteenth century, the century of the Enlightenment, that the West adopted a method of protection against smallpox that had been practiced in the East for many centuries. This method was variolation, an inoculation with true smallpox which produces a milder attack than spontaneous infection, thus giving protection against future attacks. The West was made aware of this Eastern method for the first time by the writings of two residents of Constantinople, Emanuel Timoni (1713), a physician, and Lady Mary Wortley Montagu (1718), the wife of the British ambassador. But variolation was a dangerous method. Once medicine had accepted the practice of prevention against smallpox, a far better and safer method was evolved by Edward Jenner (1749–1823).

Jenner, a country practitioner, had heard of the immunity against smallpox enjoyed by milkmaids formerly infected by cowpox. With the encouragement of his teacher, John Hunter, he began to investigate this phenomenon. In his *Inquiry into the Causes and Effects of Variolae Vaccinae,* published in 1798, Jenner demonstrated that inoculation with cowpox would produce protection against smallpox in man without ill effects to the patient. The method, called vaccination, spread rapidly and has been of incalculable benefit to mankind. It has reduced the occurrence of smallpox to such an extent that the politically inclined World Health Organization found it possible to announce the "eradication" of smallpox. This announcement might be premature in view of the unreliability of statistics in underdeveloped countries.

Yet another effect of the Enlightenment, and the resulting philanthropic trend, was the revival of interest in medical ethics. Thomas Percival's *Code of Ethics,* published in Manchester, one of the first modern industrial towns, in 1803, became the model for all later codes. Doctors in the eighteenth century enjoyed such high social standing and such high emoluments that later generations have looked upon this period as the Golden Age of the medical profession. The relatively small number of doctors were usually attached to the courts of princes or to the freely spending families of the privileged aristocracy. In the speculation on how larger groups could be provided with medical care, insurance schemes and plans for university reforms appeared.

A child of the eighteenth century is the homeopathic system of Samuel Hahnemann (1755–1843). Hahnemann's system involved the use of infinitesimally small doses of such drugs as would produce the symptoms of the disease when given in large doses. The system is summed up in the phrase, *Similia similibus curantur* (Like is cured by like). This theory has not been confirmed by scientific experience, but it was probably no more erroneous than any of the other eighteenth-century systems, and it became very popular in the early nineteenth century. At least Hahnemann's system offered a fairly innocuous alternative to the heroic and often fatal orthodox therapeutic methods of the age, which still consisted of extensive bloodletting, purging, large doses of toxic drugs, and induced vomiting. The dogmatism of his system has separated it from the main stream of scientific development, and it now lives on as a cult with a relatively small following. The other medical heresy of the late eighteenth century, Mesmer's "animal magnetism," will be dealt with later in relation to the growth of psychiatry. Both Hahnemann and Mesmer were freemasons.

Chapter 12

THE CLINICAL SCHOOLS
OF THE FIRST HALF OF THE
NINETEENTH CENTURY

Medicine had been scientific in intention for a long time. But only during the nineteenth century did it become to a large extent scientific in fact. In general it was the systematic promotion and application of natural science which gave the nineteenth century its most characteristic features. This is not the place to present a detailed discussion of nineteenth-century trends. But the reader should remember that the developments in medicine, in technology, and in science during this period were paralleled in economics by the growth of industry and capitalism, and in politics by the evolution of democracy and nationalism.

In later decades of the nineteenth century progress in medicine was largely gained through the adaptation of the results of natural science to medical uses. But the first great step forward in scientific medicine was not achieved in this way. Medicine began by rescuing itself, like the legendary Baron von Muenchhausen who pulled himself out of a swamp by tugging on his own pigtails. The medical profession freed itself from the morass of eighteenth-century theories and systems and made a sweeping return to clinical observation, checked and complemented by extensive and intensive studies on the autopsy table. This was more than a return to Hippocratic methods. The clinical "observation" of the early nineteenth century differed in three essential points from the classical Hippocratic observation. To begin with, it was

large-scale. While the famous clinic of Boerhaave consisted
of only six beds for men and six beds for women, Bouillaud,
one of the leaders of the Paris Clinical School, could boast
of having seen twenty-five thousand cases within five years.
Furthermore, nineteenth-century clinical observation was
no longer the passive art practiced by clinicians from Hippocrates to Sydenham and Boerhaave; it was transformed into
active *examination* through the large-scale application of new
and revived methods of physical diagnosis. Finally, observation was no longer concerned with unexplained symptoms,
but with symptoms considered in the light of lesions found
at the autopsy table.

In the Middle Ages medicine had centered round libraries.
During the following three centuries, as in classical antiquity,
it had focused upon the individual sickbed. But in the nineteenth century it centered round hospitals. Hospitals were
such a decisive factor in the development of early nineteenth-
century medicine that this particular period might well be
characterized as the period of *hospital* medicine, as distinguished from its predecessors, *library* and *bedside* medicine,
and its successor, which can aptly be called *laboratory*
medicine.

Hospitals had existed before, but their number increased
prodigiously as the Industrial Revolution fostered rapid ur-
banization. Refuge had to be found for the tens of thousands
of young peasants, male and female, who were streaming
into the growing cities. All too often they fell victims to
typhoid fever or tuberculosis, diseases which as a result are
found to be in the center of the clinical interests of the period.
The new arrivals, having neither homes nor families to take
care of them, became hospital patients. The crowded hospital offered unprecedented material for clinical observation
—and for autopsies. No difficulties stood in the way of secur-
ing autopsy permits in the case of these socially uprooted
masses.

France, particularly Paris, was the starting point for this
new type of medicine, and it was in the hospitals of Paris

that it reached its climax. The political situation in Paris was conducive to change. The Revolution had abolished all the old universities, academies, and other traditional institutions. When the medical school, l'Ecole de Santé, was opened in Paris in 1794, French medicine had been freed from the grip of tradition which had stifled it for so long. New departures were easier here than in any other European country.

The politicians of the French Revolution had been profoundly influenced by the philosophers of Enlightenment. The medical revolutionaries were no less influenced by philosophers, especially by Pierre Jean Georges Cabanis (1757–1808). Cabanis, a freemason, was an Idéologue, or sensualist, who believed in the primacy of sense impressions and therefore stressed the predominant importance of clinical observation. Through his influence, French medical education was rebuilt primarily on clinical grounds. The most prominent clinician of the first twenty years of the Paris Clinical School was another Idéologue, Philippe Pinel, mentioned in the last chapter as a psychiatrist and philanthropist. It was Pinel who suggested to his pupil, Marie François Xavier Bichat (1771–1802), that he look for the seat of certain diseases in particular tissues of the body. This suggestion started Bichat on his epoch-making work on tissues. The idea was first put forward in 1788 by J. C. Smythe (1741–1821).

To Bichat the ultimate unit in physiology was not the organ, as it had been to Morgagni, but the tissue, of which he described twenty-one kinds. Instead of referring simply to inflammation of the heart, he thought in terms of pericarditis, myocarditis, and endocarditis. As much an experimenter as a dissector, Bichat integrated his anatomical studies into a vitalist physiological system. The main effect of his work was to strengthen localistic and solidistic tendencies and to bolster interest in pathological anatomy—his was the pronouncement that "Several autopsies will give you more light than twenty years of observation of symptoms." Bichat's

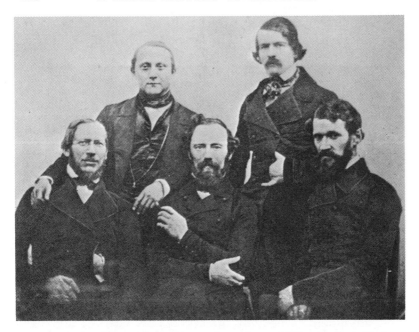

FIGURE 15. Virchow and Keolliker in Wuerzburg, 1850 (*standing*, Virchow left, Keolliker right; *sitting*, Scherer, Kiwisch, Rinecker).

tragic early death, probably from tuberculosis, prevented him from establishing the new clinical medicine on a firm foundation. And his teacher, Pinel, was unable to assume this lead. Despite all his modernistic insights, Pinel was essentially a man of the eighteenth century, still primarily interested in classifying diseases on the basis of symptoms and still adhering to such mysterious notions as "essential fevers," the description of which fills one-third of his famous *Nosographie Philosophique* (1798).

The radical break with the past was actually brought about by another pupil of Pinel, François Joseph Victor Broussais (1772–1838), a former Napoleonic soldier and a prominent liberal. His manifesto of 1816, *Examen de la doctrine médicale généralement adoptée,* attacked Pinel in an unrestrained fashion. Through Broussais essentialism was buried, and localism was made the law. The medicine of symptoms was transformed into a medicine of lesions. The artificial creation of disease units, so dear to the systematists,

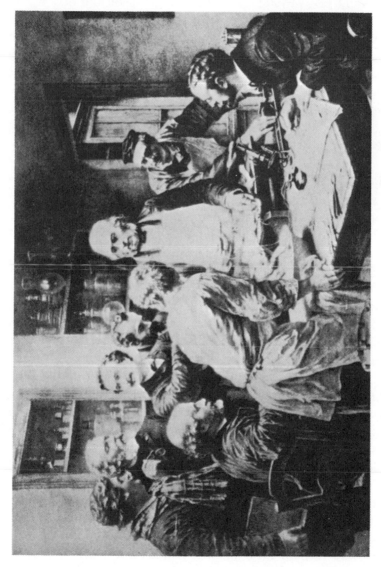

FIGURE 16. Claude Bernard surrounded by his pupils (painting by L'Hermitte).

was condemned as "ontology." The brilliant and aggressive Broussais became immensely popular in a short time. Unfortunately his "physiological medicine," as he dubbed it, degenerated into yet another system. Influenced by his numerous dissections of cases of typhoid fever, he was led to limit his pathology more and more to lesions of the gastro-intestinal tract. This oversimplification affected his therapeutic methods, and finally he settled almost exclusively on treatment by means of leeches and diet. Reflecting his influence, France imported no less than forty-two million leeches in 1833.

The essence of the teaching of the Paris Clinical School—the combination of physical examination and autopsy as the basis of clinical medicine—had in fact already been presented in Pinel's time in a much purer form by Jean Nicolas Corvisart (1755–1821), the body physician of Napoleon. Corvisart was an early exponent of bedside teaching and left an excellent treatise on the diseases of the heart. Corvisart's translation, published in 1808, of Auenbrugger's *Inventum Novum* finally made the latter's discovery generally known and accepted. While Pinel had, not accidentally, translated British material, Corvisart preferred Viennese authors.

It was through the work of Corvisart's pupils, Gaspard Laurent Bayle (1774–1816) and René Théophile Hyacinthe Laennec (1781–1826), that auscultation was added to the existing techniques of physical diagnosis. Bayle, who left a valuable book on phthisis, a disease from which he himself died young, made a beginning in the practice of direct auscultation. Stimulated by this, his younger friend Laennec invented the stethoscope and indirect or mediate auscultation (1819). Laennec thereby did more than provide the medical profession with a somewhat more dignified symbol than the medieval urinal; he opened a whole new world for medicine. His clinical and pathological descriptions of pulmonary tuberculosis in his immortal treatise on the diseases of the chest—he himself died from tuberculosis at the age of forty-five—are unsurpassed. He united all the dissimilar manifestations of this disease into one consistent pathological concept. He described for the first time such conditions as bronchiectasis, pneumothorax, hemorrhagic pleurisy, pulmonary gangrene, infarct, and emphysema.

Laennec is today considered the greatest of the French clinicians and one of the great clinicians of all times. But he enjoyed little popularity during his lifetime, partially because of his extreme Royalism. He was never able to overthrow Broussais' leadership. This task was left to other members of his circle, known as the "pathological anatomical school." One of the first to challenge Broussais' position was Gabriel Andral (1791–1876). Andral's critical clinics earned him contemporary fame, and his interest in blood chemistry marks him as a pioneer of the later laboratory medicine.

Broussais' authority was probably undermined most effectively by Pierre Charles Alexandre Louis (1787–1872), the inventor of the numerical method, otherwise known as clinical statistics. In his painstaking books on tuberculosis and typhoid fever (the latter term is his), Louis tried to determine by statistical methods the main symptoms of these diseases and the lesions corresponding to them. Also very effective were Louis' statistical inquiries into the effect of bloodletting, which showed that this panacea of Broussais and earlier authors was in many cases useless, if not detrimental. Paris was at this time the Mecca of medical students of all nations, and Louis was the teacher of numerous American graduate students, including Oliver Wendell Holmes, W. W. Gerhard, and H. I. Bowditch.

It is impossible to enumerate all the outstanding Paris clinicians of the period, but mention must be made of a few. Broussais' pupil Jean-Baptiste Bouillaud (1796–1881) made a start toward the localization of aphasia and connected polyarthritis with endocarditis. He lives on in the works of Balzac as Dr. Bianchon. Pierre Adolphe Piorry (1794–1879) invented the plessimeter and mediate percussion. Pierre François Olive Rayer (1793–1867), who wrote monumental treatises on skin and kidney diseases in the classic style of the Paris Clinical School, was at the same time a forerunner of the new laboratory era in medicine. Noteworthy among his pioneering efforts were his experimental work on glanders, his founding of the *Société de Biologie,* and his sponsorship of young scientists like Claude Bernard, Davaine, and Ville-min. The younger members of the Paris School were called "eclectics," since they no longer observed the strict party lines laid down during the lives of Laennec and Broussais.

One of the most original figures of French medicine in this period was a provincial, Pierre Bretonneau (1771–1862) of Tours, who more than any of his contemporaries emphasized the specificity of diseases. Bretonneau's excellent early trea-tise on typhoid fever preceded that of Louis, but he unfor-tunately bestowed on the disease the unpronounceable name of dothienenteritis. Bretonneau also established the modern notion of diphtheria, then a very widespread and deadly dis-ease among children, and gave it its present name. He was the first to treat it by tracheotomy. Unlike most of his col-leagues, Bretonneau regarded both diseases as contagious and wrestled with the problem of immunity. The results of Bretonneau's work were made accessible to Paris medical circles by his brilliant pupil, Armand Trousseau (1801–1867). At the time of Trousseau's death, international leadership in medicine passed from French to German hands.

Surgery had an important formative influence on the Paris School. The surgeon Desault established clinical teach-ing in Paris, and Bichat, Récamier, Laennec, Cruveilhier, and Broussais were all originally trained as surgeons. While localism was thus to a certain extent brought into medicine by surgeons, the localistic orientation of medicine was in turn very stimulating to surgery. This period saw the first extirpations of the thyroid gland by Roux, of the uterus by Récamier, and of the rectum by Lisfranc. A. Lembert de-veloped intestinal sutures. The work of the great Paris clinicians was thus paralleled by the masterly exploits of French surgeons. The greatest of them all was Guillaume Dupuytren (1777–1835), originally a pathological anatomist. The chief surgeon of Napoleon's armies, Dominique Jean

Larrey (1766–1842), should be mentioned, and also Velpeau, Malgaigne, Nelaton, and Delpech. One of the great contributions of the French Revolution was the abolition of the separation between physicians and surgeons and the consequent creation of a united medical profession. How well surgery and medicine merged in the French School is evidenced by the fact that some of the outstanding surgeons of the period were equally outstanding as physicians. In this category are Lallemand, Menière, and Velpeau.

Another characteristic aspect of the Paris Clinical School, an aspect largely conditioned by its localism, was the development of specialties. According to Bichat this development was a "natural law." In a school where so much emphasis was placed on pathological anatomy it was natural that this field should become a specialty. The first professor of pathological anatomy at Paris was Jean Cruveilhier (1791–1874). Also important were the Paris dermatologists and syphilologists of the period. The development of psychiatry as a new specialty in Paris under Pinel and his eminent pupils, especially Esquirol, has already been mentioned. Pediatrics, which profited greatly from the new examination methods, had many adepts. A classic in this field is the treatise of Charles Michel Billard (1800–1832). Geriatrics was a recognized specialty, and otology developed under Itard and Menière. Legal medicine was particularly brilliant under Orfila. France gradually assumed leadership in public hygiene during this period through the work of Villermé, Fodéré, and Parent-Duchatelet. The increased emphasis on preventive medicine was due in part to a loss of confidence in the available active therapeutic methods.

It was natural that Franz Joseph Gall (1758–1828), forced to leave Austria because of his "materialism," found a refuge and a following in Paris. Gall tried to localize mental functions and diseases in the brain and attempted to diagnose such localizations from the outside by what he called "cranioscopy." He thus followed the pattern established by the Paris clinicians in seeking new local methods of physical diagnosis. His use of comparative anatomy made him the more popular in a city where this discipline flourished under Cuvier, Lamarck, and Geoffroy St. Hilaire. While his premature findings laid the foundations of the pseudoscientific cult of phrenology, his basic principles served as an important stimulus to later scientific progress.

The methods of the French Clinical School found their first application abroad in the great hospitals of Dublin, where medicine at this time went through a unique period of growth. The name of the greatest of the Dublin physicians, Robert Graves (1796–1853), is still remembered as the eponym of Graves' disease. The name of William Stokes (1804–1878), after Graves the leader of the Dublin School, is commemorated in the Stokes-Adams' syndrome (the heart block) and in the Cheyne-Stokes type of respiration. "Corrigan's pulse" is a reminder of the classic descriptions of aortic insufficiency by D. J. Corrigan (1802–1880). Counting the pulse with a watch became a routine procedure mainly through the efforts of the Dublin School. The greatest surgeon of the Dublin School was Abraham Colles of "Colles' fracture" fame.

Most of the men who represented the new hospital medicine in England were active at Guy's Hospital in London. The most important contribution of Richard Bright (1781–1858) was the connection of certain types of dropsy with albuminuria and pathological changes in the kidney (Bright's disease). Thomas Addison (1783–1860) described pernicious anemia and the syndrome, based on changes in the suprarenals, that is named for him. Thomas Hodgkin (1798–1864), a Quaker philanthropist and a pupil of Laennec, discovered what is now called Hodgkin's disease. He was primarily a pathological anatomist. In England, as in France, the clinical school was paralleled by a flourishing surgical school, whose leaders included Sir Astley Cooper, the Bell brothers, John and Charles, Benjamin Collins Brodie, William Ferguson, and James Syme, the teacher of Lord Lister.

The new clinical medicine was eventually brought to Vienna, and the New Vienna School became as famous as the Old Vienna School of van Swieten and Stoll. It is no accident that Austria was the first of the Germanic countries to accept the new trend. In spite of its political conservatism at that time, Austria was by far the richest and most powerful of the German countries. The two most famous leaders of the New Vienna School were Josef Skoda (1805–1881) and Karl Rokitansky (1804–1878). Rokitansky was the greatest pathological anatomist of his time. Skoda developed auscultation and percussion along exact physical lines. Objective examination of therapeutics had made the French clinicians skeptics. The Viennese went even one step further; some of them became "therapeutic nihilists," holding that no treatment was better than any of the then existing treatments. And they were sometimes able to prove it. Such an attitude was in the long run untenable, but it had a sobering effect on what remained for a long time medicine's weakest field. The finest accomplishments of the New Vienna School lay in the realm of specialties. Vienna excelled in the application of the new approach to dermatology, syphilology, legal medicine, and the diseases of the eye, ear, nose, and throat. The specialist Semmelweis (see Chapter 16) is probably the most typical representative of the New Vienna School both in his talents and in his limitations.

Clinical work in Germany during this period was of very low quality. Isolated advances were made in nosography, such as the description of poliomyelitis by Jacob von Heine in 1840 and the description of botulism by the romanticist Justinus Kerner in 1820. But German medicine as a whole during the first decades of the nineteenth century was under the spell of romantic natural philosophy. While British and French medicine made progress through sober observation, German physicians, under the leadership of the philosopher Schelling, indulged in extensive speculations on the essence of life and disease, on the polarities, and on paracelsian analogies between macrocosm and microcosm. The first man to introduce the new scientific methods into Germany and to teach his clinics in his mother tongue was Johann Lucas Schoenlein (1793–1864). Schoelein had started as a natural philosopher. He passed through the natural history school, which cultivated classificatory systems based on symptoms. Completing the circle, he ended by applying and teaching exact diagnostic methods with great success. He was to discover one of the first known disease-producing parasites, the *Achorion schoenleini,* a fungus that today bears his name.

Romanticism had a less deleterious effect on biological research in Germany. Important contributions were made by such outstanding men as the embryologist Ignaz Doellinger (1770–1841) and Johann Friedrich Meckel (1781–1833), pathologist and comparative anatomist, often known as the "German Cuvier." By the nature of things German surgery was best able to resist the romantic influence. During this period it can boast of a number of eminent surgeons, often foreign-trained, including the elder Langenbeck, von Walther, and the orthopedic surgeon Stromeyer. The elder von Graefe and Dieffenbach were outstanding plastic surgeons.

The history of the clinical schools during the first half of the nineteenth century in Paris, Dublin, London, and Vienna is one of the greatest chapters in medical history, and its lessons should never be forgotten. Yet the possibilities of its two basic contributions, physical diagnosis and gross pathological anatomy, were limited. Neither teaching nor research could forever be located exclusively in the wards of a hospital. Localism was a progressive movement, but it was far from providing an answer to all the problems of pathology. An inevitable dead end was reached. New ways had to be found; and they were found in the application of the basic sciences to the problems of clinical medicine.

Chapter 13

THE BASIC SCIENCES DURING THE NINETEENTH CENTURY

Before proceeding with the history of clinical medicine, it is necessary to pause and review the great advances made in the basic sciences—microscopic anatomy, physiology, pathology, and pharmacy—in the first half of the nineteenth century. By the middle of the century the exclusive use of clinical observation and autopsy, the two pillars of hospital medicine, had achieved all of which it was capable. Future progress depended on the ability of medical men to apply the great discoveries of science to their own special field.

Beginning with the nineteenth century, progress in science largely depended on the rise of a new type of scientist. Up to this time research had been in the hands of practicing physicians or wealthy amateurs. In the long run this social situation was to prove an obstacle, and future advance depended to a large extent on the development of a climate of opinion and a social milieu favorable to a new type of full-time, "pure" scientist. The reformed German universities—Germany managed to modernize her universities without a revolution—proved to be the environment in which such a development could first be realized, and the leading role of Germany in medicine during the second half of the nineteenth century is largely due to this factor. Antidissection feelings, expressed in grave-robbing scandals, still plagued the Anglo-Saxon countries. On the Continent such feelings had long ceased to interfere with medical research.

On the threshold of this new period stands the physiologist Johannes Mueller (1801–1858). A romantic in his youth, he turned exact scientist in his more mature years. During his years in Berlin he taught many of the heroes of the coming generation and was an inspiration to many more. When Mueller began his career, science was still sufficiently undeveloped to allow him to handle several disciplines at the same time. By the time of his death, the great increase in knowledge had made specialization unavoidable, and several men had to be appointed to fill the chairs he had held alone. In his universality Mueller was the last of the great naturalists of the type of Malpighi, Spallanzani, Haller, and Alexander von Humboldt. Mueller is best remembered as a physiologist. He confirmed the Bell-Magendie law and enunciated the Law of Specific Nerve Energy, which states that stimulation of the optic, acoustic, sensory, or motor nerves will always produce only optic, acoustic, sensory, or motor responses. But no less remarkable was his work in microscopic anatomy, especially on glands; in embryology, where he named the Muellerian duct; in pathological anatomy, where his work on tumors foreshadowed the cellular method and inspired the research of his pupil Virchow in this field; and in the comparative anatomy of marine fauna. Among Mueller's pupils were the histologists Schwann, Henle, Gerlach, Schulze, and Koelliker, the pathologist Virchow, and the physiologists Helmholtz, Du Bois-Reymond, Bruecke, Pflueger, and Bidder.

The numerous discoveries in histology were finally made meaningful by the cell theory. Since the beginning of the century medical scientists such as Oken and Meckel, and later Raspail, Dutrochet, and others, had claimed that living bodies consisted basically of "vesicles," "cells," or "globules." This was an advancement beyond Bichat's tissue theory. The conviction was particularly strongly held by botanists like Mirbel, Treviranus, and von Mohl. This was natural enough, since cellular structure is most easily seen in plants. In fact it was in describing plants that Robert Hooke had coined the expression "cell" in 1665. Direct knowledge of cells increased tremendously after 1830, when better microscopes were introduced, through the work of such men as Purkinjé, Valentin, and Donné.

The formulation of the cell theory was crystallized through the efforts of Theodor Schwann (1809–1885), a pupil of Johannes Mueller. Stimulated by the work of his botanist friend, Matthias Schleiden, Schwann in 1838 announced his famous theory that all living structures consisted of cells. The Schleiden-Schwann cell theory still had one very serious shortcoming, which especially hampered its applications in pathology. According to Schleiden and Schwann, cells arose from an amorphous protein mass called blastema. That cells developed from cells, and only from cells, was demonstrated by Hugo von Mohl, John Goodsir, Robert Remak, and preeminently by Rudolf Virchow in 1854. This great biological discovery, so hard to achieve with the rudimentary microscope of the time, brought to completion the cell theory which became the foundation of all modern biological thought.

Probably no microscopist of the century was the equal of Jacob Henle (1809–1885) in the discovery and description of micro-anatomic structures. Garrison likens his role in microscopy to the role of Vesalius in gross anatomy. As one of the founders of the *Zeitschrift fuer rationalle Medizin* (see Chapter 14) Henle was also a leading figure of the new era in clinical medicine. In addition, he was one of the few defenders of the theory that epidemics were produced by micro-organisms transmitted through contagion. This old theory of Fracastorius was almost completely discredited in Henle's time, but it was later to be proved true by Pasteur and Henle's own pupil, Robert Koch. Outstanding both as a microscopist and as an experimental physiologist was the Czech patriot Johannes Evangelista Purkinje (1787–1869), who was the first to use the microtome and to describe the ciliary movements in cells. His name has become an eponym for certain structures in the cerebellum. Purkinje introduced the term "protoplasm" and pointed out the importance of fingerprints for identification purposes.

Albert von Koelliker (1817–1905), author of the first formal textbook on histology, is particularly remembered for his work on the smooth muscle and the spermatozoon. He introduced the cell theory into embryology in 1844. In 1856 Augustus Volney Waller (1816–1870) introduced the use of nerve degeneration into the study of the nervous pathways. This was extremely important for the extension of this most difficult field of microscopic anatomy. In 1882 Walter Flemming elucidated the mechanism of cell division. Wilhelm Waldeyer (1837–1921) synthesized earlier work in neuroanatomy into the neuron theory in 1891. Waldeyer also proved that cancerous (carcinoma) cells stem from epithelial rather than connective tissues. He named the chromosome and did much for a better understanding of the tonsils.

Progress in histology was to a large extent dependent on the construction of better microscopes and the introduction of staining methods. As long as histologists had to work exclusively with fresh preparations, a great many of the facts now known to first-year medical students could not be discovered. Among those who introduced new staining methods were von Gerlach, Max Schultze, the pathologist Carl Weigert, and his cousin Paul Ehrlich.

Embryology is almost inseparable from histology, and progress in the two fields was interdependent. In 1821, J. L. Prévost of Geneva and J. B. Dumas, the mentor of Louis Pasteur, published a series of most important discoveries (origin of spermatozoa, place of fertilization, segmentation of the fertilized egg, and so on). Karl Ernst von Baer (1792–1876) extended the field of comparative embryology beyond the study of the chick embryo, which had been almost its sole concern since the time of Aristotle. He was the first to describe the mammalian ovum in 1827. The female sex cell thus became known almost two hundred years later than the male sex cell. Von Baer also differentiated germ layers, the concept of which was brought into its present form by Remak. The elder Wilhelm His (1831–1904) did much to trace the embryological origins of tissues and worked on the reconstruction of embryos through serial sections. Experimental embryology was introduced by Wilhelm Roux (1850–1924) in 1883.

The first great experimental physiologist of the nineteenth century was François Magendie (1783–1855). It is typical of the French orientation that Magendie functioned simultaneously as a clinician and was never professor in a medical school. Magendie exhibited in a most concentrated form the aversion of the nineteenth-century scientist from any sort of theorizing and larger synthesis. His main goal was to collect as many experimental data as possible in every field, without regard to whether they concerned the physiology of the heart, stomach, lymphatics, or central nervous system. He is best remembered for his discovery of the motor and sensory character of the anterior and posterior spinal roots, respectively. This discovery involved him in a bitter controversy over priority with Sir Charles Bell (1774–1842), the surgeon-anatomist. Another outstanding French neurophysiologist of the era was M. P. J. Flourens (1794–1867), who with his *noeud vital* in the medulla oblongata gave the first definite description of the respiratory center, observed previously by Legallois. Flourens' finest work was done in the eighteen twenties on the function of the cerebellum and the semicircular canals. He, too, was never professor on a medical faculty. Marshall Hall (1798–1857) established the concepts of unconscious reflex (dimly perceived by Willis, Bohn, and Whytt) and traumatic shock. Sir Charles Bell greatly elucidated the functions and composition of the fifth and seventh cranial nerves. It is typical of England at that time that the three greatest British physiologists—Hall, Waller, and Bowman—had to make their livings as practitioners.

Gall's theories on localization of functions in the cortex had been ridiculed, and the specific work on the speech center by his follower Bouillaud had been ignored. Only in

1861, when the great French surgeon and anthropologist Paul Broca (1824–1880) described a speech center in the region previously explored by Gall and Bouillaud, was the idea accepted. A whole new range was thus opened for localization studies. In the eighteen seventies Fritsch, Hitzig, and Ferrier mapped out the sensory and motor areas of the brain. Broca himself carried out the first practical applications of the localization principle to brain surgery. F. L. Goltz (1834–1902) made his important studies on shock in the sixties and on decerebrated animals in the seventies.

A great deal of physiological progress in the nineteenth century centered in Germany, where apparatus developed by physicists was judiciously used in physiological experiments. This trend is clearly illustrated by the work of the three Weber brothers, and the importance of it is too often not sufficiently realized. Wilhelm Eduard Weber (1804–1891) was a great physicist and contributed much to the invention of the electric telegraph. The physiologist Ernst Heinrich Weber (1795–1878) established the notion of the threshold, and was a sworn enemy of Romanticism. Together with his brother, Eduard Friedrich Weber (1806–1871), he measured the velocity of the pulse wave and demonstrated the inhibitory function of the vagus. The Weber brothers thus became the fathers of the notion of inhibition in neurophysiology.

During the 1840's four young German physiologists, Emil Du Bois-Reymond (1818–1896), Hermann Helmholtz (1821–1894), Ernst Bruecke (1819–1892), and Carl Ludwig (1816–1895), banded together to create a new and strictly scientific physiology. Although they did not reach this goal, their contribution is a tremendous one. Du Bois-Reymond laid the foundations of modern electrophysiology, while Helmholtz made many applications of physics to physiology and eventually became a pure physicist. In 1847 Helmholtz formulated the Law of the Conservation of Energy, only a few years after the formulations of Robert Mayer and Joule in 1842. As a physiologist, he measured the heat production of the muscle and the velocity of the nerve impulse. He did basic work in the physiology of the senses, in the course of which he invented the ophthalmoscope (1851), and developed the basic notions underlying the field of acoustics. Ludwig's work was devoted primarily to the physiology of the heart and circulation. Many of his finest discoveries were published as the doctoral theses of his pupils. A teacher so unselfish and disinterested was bound to attract a great number of pupils. Some of these students, men like W. H. Welch, H. P. Bowditch, F. P. Mall, and J. J. Abel, were to rejuvenate American medicine.

Most of the research reported above was carried out along physical lines with physical apparatus. The great progress of chemistry around the turn of the century made it possible for this discipline to make equally important contributions to physiology. In the twentieth century it was eventually to overshadow physical methods of research. Significantly, most of the important routine urine tests, such as those evolved by Heller, Fehling, Trommer, Pettenkofer, and Bence Jones, were developed in the eighteen forties or later. The great chemist Justus von Liebig (1803–1873) made an important contribution to human physiology through his classification of the basic foodstuffs into carbohydrates, proteins, and fats. The analysis of carbohydrates was largely due to Proust, and that of fats to Chevreul. The idea of measuring the protein metabolism by determination of the nitrogen in the urine was another contribution of Liebig's. The synthesis of an organic compound, urea, by his friend Wöhler in 1828 was of basic theoretical importance. It killed the romantic idea that "organic" chemistry has its own laws.

A pupil of Liebig, Carl von Voit (1831–1908), in collaboration with Max von Pettenkofer (1818–1901), developed the determination of basic metabolism to unprecedented heights. Voit's school had a vigorous offshoot in the United States through the influence of Dubois, Benedict, and Atwater. Voit's work was completed by his pupil Max Rubner (1854–1932), who discovered that metabolism is proportional to the surface of the body. Rubner also determined the specific dynamic action of food in metabolism, which had previously been studied by J. B. A. Chauveau. These metabolic studies made possible the introduction of a new scientific dietetics into medicine. Up to this time dietetics had been entirely empirical.

A new chapter in the understanding of digestion had opened with the discovery of the enzyme pepsin by Schwann in 1833. It was in the field of digestion, and especially with regard to the functions of the pancreatic juice, that Claude Bernard (1813–1878), a pupil of Magendie, made some of his finest discoveries. Bernard had started out as a playwright, but he was persuaded by a commendable art critic to devote his talents to medicine. Bernard coined the term "internal secretion," now used in a slightly different sense, on the occasion of his discovery of the glycogen-forming function of the liver. This discovery showed for the first time that the body plays a synthesizing role in the metabolic process as well as a decomposing one. In the course of his glycogen studies Bernard was able to produce artificial diabetes by puncture of a certain region of the fourth ventricle. One of Bernard's greatest achievements in the field of physiology was his clarification of the function and nature of the vasomotor nerves. The vasomotor system was to him an important factor in creating what he called the "internal environment," the condition that allows the relative independence of warm-blooded animals from external influences.

When illness made it necessary for Bernard to forego experimental work, he turned to theoretical writings. He synthesized the basic philosophical ideas of the nineteenth-century physiologists in his famous *Introduction to Experimental Medicine*, published in 1865. This unsurpassed manifesto has perhaps done more than anything else to make Bernard the symbol of nineteenth-century physiology. Posthumous publication of some of Bernard's notebooks has shown that his book was the well-considered outgrowth of lifelong meditations and internal conflicts carefully hidden under a mask of Olympian grandeur. Bernard still had difficulties with antivivisection feelings, but they were nothing compared with those plaguing researchers in Anglo-Saxon countries to this very day.

Another great experimenter of the nineteenth century, Charles Edouard Brown-Séquard (1817–1894), was born of an American father and a French mother in the island of Mauritius and was active in the United States, France, and England. Though he was always overshadowed by Bernard during the latter's lifetime, he preceded the latter in the discovery of the vasomotor nerves. It was Brown-Séquard who opened the era of gland therapy and large-scale interest in endocrinology. In 1889 he experimented on himself with testicular extracts and rejuvenated himself to the extent that he acquired the whooping cough at the age of seventy-two. Experimental work in endocrinology, by such men as A. A. Berthold, M. Schiff, and Brown-Séquard himself, dates back to the eighteen forties and eighteen fifties. But it became of practical importance only after Brown-Séquard's experiments in the eighteen eighties. The studies of Paul Bert (1830–1886), the favorite pupil of Claude Bernard, on the physiological effects of changes in barometric pressure, including the effects of hypotension as well as hypertension, were of fundamental importance for aviation physiology. In fact, his book, written in 1878, had to be translated into English during the Second World War for practical purposes.

Physiological chemistry became a separate discipline under the leadership of Felix Hoppe-Seyler (1825–1895), a pupil of Rudolf Virchow, whose career seemed so hopeless in its beginning that he decided to emigrate to the United States and almost did so. His outstanding work was done in the field of blood chemistry. He discovered hemoglobin in 1862.

In 1846 the great Rokitansky, at that time undisputed leader in the field of pathological anatomy, published the first volume of his *Handbook of General Pathological Anatomy*. Not satisfied with his extensive localistic work, he tried to create a synthetic theory of pathology in the form of a doctrine of "dyscrasias." But unfortunately his factual foundation was insufficient, and the only result was a relapse into speculative humoral pathology. The theory was completely demolished in a review by a young Berlin pathologist, Rudolf Virchow (1821–1902), and in subsequent editions of the book Rokitansky did not reprint the disputed passages.

Virchow had already attracted the attention of the medical profession by his discovery of leukemia and his experimental studies on embolism and thrombosis, both of which terms were coined by him. In these studies he disproved Cruveilhier's oversimplified derivation of all diseases from phlebitis. It must be remembered that this preoccupation with inflammation of the veins was natural enough in a period when the pathological material was largely drawn from cases of wound gangrene and puerperal fever. Virchow symbolizes the shift from gross to miscroscopical anatomy in the pathological field. During the following decades he was to enrich pathology with hundreds of detailed studies. He discovered amyloid, hematoidin, and myelin; he worked on connective tissues and inflammation; and he studied tumors (1863) and trichinosis (1864). But even more important than these individual contributions was his establishment of the basic principles which since his day have reigned supreme in pathological anatomy. In his *Cellular Pathology,* published in 1858, one year before Darwin's *Origin of Species,* he showed that the cell is the ultimate unit of pathological disturbances as well as of normal life. By the use of this criterion it was possible to bring order to an overwhelming mass of detailed facts. Virchow's demonstration that every cell is the product of another cell was a very important contribution to general biology. It is interesting to note that the cellular theory as a basic theory of pathology was developed almost simultaneously with the atomic theory as the basic theory of physics.

During the second half of the nineteenth century Virchow became the best known and the most respected medical man of his time, a kind of "Pope" of medicine. It is significant of the spirit of the times that this role of leadership was now assumed by a laboratory man. Virchow was by no means infallible, and this overwhelming position of his occasionally led to the propagation of misconceptions, as happened in the case of his views on tuberculosis and diphtheria. On the other hand he has been unjustly accused of lack of understanding of the new bacteriology and the new evolutionary theories. A reading of Virchow's polemics against his ex-pupils Klebs and Haeckel leads one to feel that he was only defending sound scientific skepticism against dangerous enthusiasms.

Virchow's laboratory work did not isolate him from society. His participation in the 1848 revolution cost him his position in Berlin, so that from 1849 to 1856 he taught in Wuerzburg. After his return to Berlin he was the leader of the liberal opposition in Prussia during the decisive sixties until he was defeated by Bismarck. During the last thirty years of his life, Virchow's creative work was devoted almost exclusively to anthropology and archeology, and he must be regarded as one of the founders of these disciplines. Naturally, Virchow was also greatly interested in public health. He regarded his report on the 1848 typhus epidemic in Upper Silesia as the decisive event in his life. His social theory of epidemics and his dictum, "Medicine is a social science," are well remembered. The transformation of Berlin into a healthy city was largely his work.

Among the many gifted pupils of Virchow were Hoppe-Seyler, already mentioned, and the pathologists Friedrich Daniel von Recklinghausen (1833–1910) and Julius Cohnheim (1839–1884). The latter elucidated the cellular mechanism of inflammation by demonstrating the migration of the leukocytes through the wall of the vessel. Virchow himself had believed in the local formation of the leukocyte in inflammation. The fact that his pupil thus destroyed one of the master's main theories shows that Virchow was by no means the stubborn tyrant he has sometimes been called.

Drug treatment had so far been purely empirical. The successes of the experimental method in physiology, combined with the spectacular progress of chemical analysis, naturally led to the application of these methods to the examination of drugs. Thus a new science, pharmacology, was born. It is no accident that Magendie, a leading physiologist, was one of the fathers of modern pharmacology. Modern pharmacology was possible only after the pharmacists had isolated sufficiently pure substances from the raw drugs. The first substances thus to be isolated were in the alkaloid family. Sertuerner isolated morphine in 1806, and Pelletier and Caventou did the same for strychnine in 1818 and quinine in 1820. Magendie worked with strychnine, morphine, emetine, the bromides, and iodine. His pupil Bernard analyzed opium, nicotine, ether, and curare. In Germany, pharmacology became an independent discipline through Rudolf Buchheim (1820–1879). His pupil Oswald Schmiedeberg (1838–1921) did important research, especially on digitalis and histamine. He became the founder of a school which spread all over the world. In England Alexander Crum Brown and Thomas Frazer (1841–1920) related chemical constitution to pharmacological effects. Sir Thomas Lauder Brunton (1844–1916) analyzed heart drugs and introduced the use of amyl nitrite for angina pectoris. During the 1880's, the rapidly growing pharmaceutical industry introduced numerous synthetic drugs. Most of these were antipyretics, such as antipyrine, salipyrin, acetanilid, and sulfonal. From this beginning there developed in the twentieth century the science of specific drugs, or chemotherapy, which will be considered in a later chapter.

The basic sciences gave medicine an unprecedented knowledge of the intricate structures of the human body. They provided a means of correlating pathological signs with changes in those structures; they allowed the main functions of the body—respiration, circulation, digestion, metabolism, nervous action, internal secretion, and reproduction—to be understood as never before; they made possible the objective measurement of these functions and their deviations from the normal; and they made therapeutic action equally predictable and measurable. It is obvious that this new background was to have a decisive influence on the future development of clinical medicine.

Chapter 14

CLINICAL MEDICINE OF THE SECOND HALF OF THE NINETEENTH CENTURY

The spectacular progress of histology, pathology, physiology, and pharmacology led to the development of a new type of clinical medicine in the second half of the nineteenth century. This new clinical medicine is the medicine of the present day. One of its early protagonists, Claude Bernard, pronounced that the laboratory was the "sanctuary" of medicine. Thus the new period can properly be called that of laboratory medicine, as opposed to the library medicine of the Middle Ages, the bedside medicine of Hippocrates, Boerhaave, and Sydenham, and the hospital medicine of Laennec and Graves. Laboratory medicine, which replaces immediate sense impressions with numbers, tends to become "abstract medicine," especially when compared with its predecessor. Germany played a leading role in the new development, since it was only in Germany that there had grown up a large body of full-time scientists. There were numerous professional physiologists and institutes of physiology in Germany, while in Great Britain, for example, research and teaching in physiology still depended mainly on the work of medical practitioners.

At about the same time that Helmholtz, Ludwig, Bruecke, and Du Bois-Reymond began their cooperation in the field of physiology, several groups of young German doctors were founding new medical journals for the purpose of creating a new clinical medicine. Wunderlich, Roser, and Griesinger started the *Journal of Physiological Medicine* in 1842; Henle and Pfeufer launched the *Journal of Rational Medicine* in 1844; and Virchow and Reinhardt established the *Archives for Pathological Anatomy, Physiology and Clinical Medicine* in 1847. As competitors in the pursuit of the same goal, these men fought one another repeatedly, but fundamentally their approach was the same. They were reacting violently against the romantic past that had led German medicine into the dead end of vain speculation. But at the same time they refused to be satisfied with the type of medicine represented by the Paris and Vienna schools. They rejected what they called the "ontological approach" of these schools; medicine should be concerned primarily with the study of disturbed function, not with the artificial construction of disease entities. The young Germans also objected to the purely anatomical approach of Paris and Vienna. They maintained that what was observed on the autopsy table was only the end result of a pathological process, not the process itself. This process could be ascertained only by a study of disturbed function. Thus "pathological physiology" became the slogan of the new school. The influence of Broussais can be seen in this approach.

The future was to show that this criticism of the ontological approach was premature. The fault of Pinel and Schoenlein lay, not in constructing disease entities as such, but in constructing wrong disease entities. The "ontological" disease entities of a Laennec or a Bretonneau have been fully confirmed by the discoveries of bacteriology. On the other hand, the stand taken by the reformers in favor of pathological physiology, as opposed to the purely anatomical approach, was sound and progressive. Just as anatomy had to develop from Vesalius to Harvey, from morphology to physiology, so the clinic had to advance from the study of pathologic structures to the study of pathologic function based on pathologic structure.

The integration of laboratory results and clinical observation was by no means an easy task—and it remains difficult today. Some time elapsed before the new type of medicine became more than an appendage of the laboratory. The early stages are well represented by the two Berlin clinicians, Friedrich Theodor von Frerichs (1819–1885), who primarily studied liver disease, and Ludwig Traube (1818–1876), who experimentally investigated pneumonia and kidney and heart diseases. The systematic study of temperature change in disease was developed to a high level by Carl Wunderlich (1815–1877) in the sixties. This was pathological physiology at its best. On the other hand, it is one of the ironies of history that Wunderlich, who had set out to fight "ontology," ended by constructing an ontology of his own with his theory of specific temperature charts for specific diseases. A consequence of Wunderlich's research was the so-called "anti-pyretic wave" in therapeutics. Fevers were now ruthlessly suppressed, especially with new drugs like salicylic acid, antipyrin, and phenacetin. One of the most representative and many-sided clinicians of the time was Adolf Kussmaul (1822–1902), who wrote on the psychology of the newborn in 1859 and on periarteritis nodosa in 1860. In 1874 he demonstrated the part played by acetonemia in the diabetic coma. His introduction of the stomach pump for the treatment of stomach disease in 1867 opened the way for the study of stomach function. The study of function grew more and more to be the creed of the new clinical medicine.

It was in this field of stomach diseases that the interest of the clinician first shifted from the study of structure to the study of function. The mobility, secretion, and digestive abilities of the stomach were now of more concern to the clinician than its postmortem morphology or the acoustic phenomena observed during life. Test meals for the study of stomach function were developed by Carl Anton Ewald (1845–1915) and Ismar Boas (1858–1938). One of the pioneers of the functional approach was Ottomar Rosenbach (1851–1907), who in the seventies claimed that function, rather than configuration, was the essential factor. Consequently he began to substitute the concept of ventricular insufficiency for that of ventricular dilatation in an attempt to replace anatomical by functional diagnosis. He coined such useful notions as that of the "latent reserve force" of organs.

The functional interest was also predominant in the studies of the cardiologist James Mackenzie (1853–1925) on the irregularities of the heart beat. The diseases of the kidney and the liver were approached in similar fashion. Although the tests for blood urea, blood bilirubin, and blood sugar are of more recent vintage, the principles underlying these tests, which essentially ascertain function, were established in the second half of the nineteenth century. Friedrich von Mueller (1858–1941) and Adolf Magnus Levy (born 1865) showed that the state of such internal-secretion glands as the thyroid could be ascertained by testing the function of metabolism. Bernhard Naunyn (1839–1925) devoted himself primarily to the study of diabetes and gallstones, and it was in his clinic in Strasbourg in 1889 that Minkowski and von Mering made the decisive experiment which proved that diabetes was due to pancreatic disease. The experiment itself—the extirpation of the pancreas in dogs—had been performed as early as 1683 by the Swiss Johann Conrad Brunner, but its consequences had not been understood. In addition to Mackenzie, typical representatives of laboratory medicine in England were Sir Thomas Clifford Allbutt (1836–1925) and the Canadian Sir William Osler (1849–1919), who was for many years active in the United States. Most of the great clinical accomplishments in England and in France in this period were in the field of neurology. They will be mentioned later when that specialty is discussed.

The use of laboratory studies in physiology, experimental pathology, and pharmacology contributed greatly to the increase of clinical knowledge, especially diagnostic knowledge. Nevertheless the results were gradual rather than dramatic. Even this new type of research rarely penetrated to the actual causes of disease, and the main therapeutic harvest of this approach was reaped only in the twentieth century. The early results were sufficient to provoke the enthusiasm of the scientifically minded physician. But to fire the imagination of the average practitioner and the layman something more dramatic, something of more immediate usefulness, had to come out of the laboratory. Only then could scientific medicine achieve its present standing.

This dramatic event was the discovery that infectious diseases are caused by micro-organisms. From this discovery grew the new science of bacteriology, or microbiology as it is usually called now, the youngest of the basic sciences. In the seventh and eighth decades of the century one organism after another was identified; vaccination, serum therapy, and preventive measures were developed in quick succession; and a start was made toward the virtual elimination of a whole group of diseases. These events gave definite proof of the value of the laboratory approach.

Chapter 15

MICROBIOLOGY

The idea that epidemic diseases were transmitted by contagion, and caused by micro-organisms, "seeds," or "animalculae," was not exactly new in the middle of the nineteenth century. The theory had been set forth by Fracastorius in the sixteenth century, and it had been defended by Kircher in the seventeenth century and by Lancisi and Linné in the eighteenth. As a matter of fact, it was at the lowest ebb in its history when Jacob Henle again proclaimed it in 1840; and he appeared to his contemporaries, not as the precursor of a new era, but as the gallant defender of an old-fashioned error. Epidemiological experience with yellow fever, typhus, and cholera, in which quarantines had proved to be supremely ineffective, supported the claims of the anticontagionists, who had in their ranks such respectable scientists as Magendie, Villermé, Bouillaud, and Corrigan. To look for a living agent of contagion was even less fashionable in a period when belief in the prospects of chemistry was almost unlimited. Thus the chemist Liebig could successfully override even such clear evidence for the role of living forms in chemical processes as that presented in favor of the fermentation through yeast by Cagniard de Latour in 1836 and Schwann and Kuetzig in 1837.

Yet in the second half of the nineteenth century medical opinion was slowly to change. This was partially a pendulumlike return to a previous position, since anticontagionism had proved to be just about as ineffective against cholera epidemics as the old-fashioned contagionism. A more positive factor was the rapidly accumulating evidence in favor of the causation of disease by micro-organisms. One of the most important steps in this direction was the demonstration by the lawyer Agostino Bassi in 1835 that certain diseases of the silkworm were contagious, being produced by fungi. Bassi drew far-reaching conclusions from these discoveries as to the nature of contagious diseases in general. In 1837 Donné demonstrated the presence of the organism *Trichomonas vaginalis;* in 1839 Schoenlein described the fungus causing favus (named after him by Remak); and David Gruby described other fungi causing skin disease in 1844.

Finally, in 1850, bacteria were added to the list of possible disease-causing micro-organisms. Bacteria had first been seen by Leeuwenhoek. They had been studied extensively by the Danish naturalist Mueller in the eighteenth century and by the naturalist Ehrenberg and the botanist Ferdinand Cohn in the nineteenth century. But so far they had not been suspected of pathogenic potentialities. Casimir Davaine (1812–1882) and Pierre Rayer (1793–1867) discovered the anthrax bacillus in 1850 in the blood of animals dying from anthrax and succeeded in transmitting it. In 1855 Pollender published the same discovery, based on observations he had made in 1849. It was no accident that the first pathogenic bacterium discovered was one of the largest. Davaine, a general practitioner, did not even have a laboratory; he kept his experimental animals in a friend's garden. Other pathogenic micro-organisms discovered during this period were the trichinae, whose pathogenic qualities were discovered by Virchow and Zenker in 1860, and the spirilla causing relapsing fever, discovered by Virchow's assistant, Obermeier, in 1868. In 1872 Coze, Feltz, and Davaine submitted extensive evidence for the bacterial causation of septicemia. The idea of contagion was supported by inoculation experiments on such diseases as glanders. The first of these was performed by Rayer in 1837. Villemin proved the contagiousness of tuberculosis by inoculation experiments in 1865. Similar experiments had been made by Klencke in 1843 without receiving recognition.

That these isolated, primarily practical observations developed into a new science is due largely to the genius of one man, Louis Pasteur (1822–1895). Pasteur, born the son of a tanner at Dole in the Jura mountains, was not a medical man but a chemist. This may explain why he approached medical problems in a basic, scientific fashion, rather than reaching out immediately for practical answers. After holding the post of chemistry professor in Dijon, Strasbourg, and Lille, Pasteur went to Paris in 1857 as director of scientific studies in the École Normale, which educated college and university professors for the whole country. It was as a chemist that in 1848 he made his first great discovery by establishing the existence of molecular dissymmetry. And it was as a chemist that he began his studies on fermentations in 1857. The results of these fermentation studies were contrary to prevailing chemical opinion, which looked upon fermentation as a purely chemical event. Pasteur showed conclusively that fermentation was the work of various micro-organisms. These findings launched Pasteur into what was to become bacteriology.*

Progress in the science of bacteria demanded the elimination of the theory of their spontaneous generation, which had still not been completely disproved. This work was accomplished by Pasteur in a series of masterly experiments in 1862. As a specialist in micro-organisms he was now widely sought by governmental and private organizations to help save French industries, menaced by processes which seemed to be the work of micro-organisms. His study of the diseases of wine led to his invention in 1863 of the process that still bears his name, "pasteurization." He studied the diseases of the silkworm in 1865 and the diseases of beer in 1871. Pasteur's successful identification of the responsible micro-organisms saved important branches of the French economy from ruin. He continued working ceaselessly, though a hemiplegic attack in 1868 left him rather handicapped.

* The term "bacteriology" is used here in the traditional, nonprecise sense as the science of *all* pathogenic micro-organisms.

Only in 1877, after twenty years of research into the biology of micro-organisms, did Pasteur extend his studies to the diseases of men and higher animals. He first attacked the problem of anthrax and chicken cholera. Not satisfied with identifying the disease-producing organisms, in 1880 he turned, with the help of such brilliant pupils as Roux, Chamberland, and Thuillier, toward the elaboration of preventive vaccines for both diseases, which had been tried before by the veterinarians Toussaint and Galtier. His great successes in these fields led him in 1885 to his most spectacular achievement, preventive vaccination against rabies. The principle of vaccination was extended in the nineties by Fraenkel to diphtheria, by Widal and Wright to typhoid fever, and by Haffkine to cholera and plague.

A grateful nation built Pasteur a special research institute in 1889, and a grateful world honored him in every possible way. Pasteur is remembered for his restless, creative genius, and for his great human kindness. Yet he possessed another quality which was no less necessary in order to bring about the victory of his ideas—his tireless ability to fight. Great ideas and great inventions do not necessarily win acceptance because of their inherent value. Pasteur's victory was the more remarkable because he not only had to overcome the traditional conservatism of the medical profession but furthermore had to achieve this as an outsider, a nonmedical man dictating in medical matters.

Inseparably linked with Pasteur in the creation of the science of bacteriology is the name of Robert Koch (1843–1910). Unlike Pasteur, Koch had a medical background, having received his medical degree at Goettingen under Henle. While a salaried physician in eastern Germany he was impelled by scientific curiosity to experiment with anthrax. His startling findings, submitted in 1876, explained many of the unknown phases of the life cycle of this bacillus. The importance of the discoveries of this unknown country physician was immediately recognized by the Breslau botanist Ferdinand Cohn and the Breslau pathologist Cohnheim, who furthered Koch's career in a most disinterested manner.

Koch used solid media and developed new methods of fixing and staining. These great improvements in technique enabled him in 1879 to identify the bacteria causing wound infection. Outstanding scientists, including Recklinghausen, Edwin Klebs, Lister, Billroth, and Hallier, had failed to solve the same problem because of the tremendous technical difficulties they had encountered in attempting to obtain pure cultures, difficulties they never overcame. They had rationalized their failures into the theory of polymorphism, which held that bacteria were able to transform themselves into different types. Polymorphism had already been criticized by Ferdinand Cohn; Koch's work completely annihilated the theory.

In an attempt to stem the wave of uncritical work that now started in bacteriology, Koch issued his famous postulates, the genesis of which can be found in the treatise on contagion written by his teacher, Henle. These postulates were: (1) The organism should be found in each case of the disease; (2) it should not be found in other diseases; (3) it should be isolated; (4) it should be cultured; (5) it should, when inoculated, produce the same disease; (6) it should be recovered from the inoculated animal.

In 1880 Koch was called to Berlin. In 1882 he discovered —simultaneously with Paul Baumgartner—the tuberculosis bacillus, and in 1883, on a trip to Egypt and India, he found the cholera bacillus. These two discoveries made possible a successful offensive against two of the most pernicious enemies of mankind. When Koch submitted his tuberculin to the medical profession in 1890, the medical world felt that it had at last found an efficient method of treating tuberculosis. This hope was not to be confirmed by experience, but tuberculin proved to be a valuable diagnostic aid. Koch's last important research was his study of the cattle plague in South Africa in 1897 and the plague itself in India in 1898.

Koch was a far less spectacular figure than Pasteur. Arriving twenty years later on the scene, he found much better conditions for his work. Yet it should be remembered that his most characteristic qualities, great industry and technical ingenuity, are essential conditions for scientific progress.

Reasons of space make it impossible to go into the details of the growth of bacteriology. After the first decisive steps were taken, the advances of the seventies and eighties were breath-taking. At the same time, of course, there was a great deal of worthless work by incompetent enthusiasts who explained every disease and every biological function in terms of bacteria. A partial list of diseases whose causative agents were discovered during the next decades, together with the names of the discoverers, illustrates the rapid rate of progress:

1875 amebic dysentery (Loesch)
1879 gonorrhea (Neisser)
1880 typhoid fever (Eberth, Gaffky)
       leprosy (Hansen)
       malaria (Laveran)
1882 tuberculosis (Koch)
       glanders (Loeffler)
1883 erysipelas (Fehleisen)
       cholera (Koch)
1884 diphtheria (Klebs, Loeffler)
       tetanus (Nikolaier, Kitasato)
       pneumonia (A. Fraenkel)
1887 epidemic meningitis (Weichselbaum)
       malta fever (Bruce)
1889 soft chancre (Ducrey)
1892 gas gangrene (Welch)
1894 plague (Yersin, Kitasato)
       botulism (van Ermengem)
1898 bacillary dysentery (Shiga)
1901 sleeping disease (Bruce, Dutton)
1905 syphilis (Schaudinn)
1906 whooping cough (Bordet)

In the 1890's it was realized by investigators, chiefly Loeffler and Roux, that a number of diseases, such as the hoof-and-mouth disease of cattle, were caused by organisms so small that they had been passing through the so-called Chamberland filters used to retain bacteria. These organisms, called filtrable viruses, were so minute that they could not be demonstrated under ordinary microscopes. A third group of organisms, occupying a position between the viruses and the bacteria, was identified in the twentieth century and called Rickettsia.

It is impossible to give biographical details on the many important pioneer bacteriologists of the nineteenth century. These men were to be found in every European country and especially in France and Germany, where the influence of Pasteur and Koch was strongest. In addition, two countries which heretofore had not made important contributions to medical science now entered the field with important bacteriological discoveries: Japan through the work of Kitasato and Shiga, and the United States through the work of Welch, Flexner, and Theobald Smith.

Most of the fundamental bacteriological discoveries were made between 1878 and 1887. Spurred by the immortal example of Pasteur, bacteriologists did not limit themselves to simple identification of disease-producing organisms. Between 1886 and 1896 they tackled serology and immunology, thus branching out into the field of therapeutics. In 1889 Yersin and Roux demonstrated that the essential damage in diphtheria was not done by the organism causing the disease, but rather by toxins produced by the organism and circulated in the blood stream. In the same year Faber made the same discovery in the case of tetanus. A year later Emil Behring (1854–1917) and Kitasato demonstrated that the body developed antitoxins for tetanus. In 1890 Behring was also able to develop effective diphtheria antitoxins which, when injected, neutralized the toxins. Thus Behring opened the door to the field of serum therapy. His discovery considerably reduced mortality from one of the most murderous children's diseases. At the same time it suggested the production of similar antitoxins for tetanus, snake bite, and other diseases. Paul Ehrlich (1854–1915) named this procedure passive immunization, as opposed to the active immunization, or vaccination, whose discovery has already been traced. Ehrlich himself did important work on antitoxins and immunity and discovered the first autoimmune disease. Serum therapy is the first important chapter in the history of modern specific therapy.

The fact that pathogenic micro-organisms produced an increase of antibodies in the blood was used for diagnostic purposes on a large scale in Widal's agglutination test for typhoid fever in 1896. This was the beginning of serum diagnosis. Later important steps in this field were the complement-fixation test of Bordet (1902) and Wassermann's syphilis test (1906). Some serologists, like Behring in his first enthusiasm, felt that their results ushered in a new era of "humoral pathology" and marked the end of cellular pathology. But the demonstration of phagocytosis by Metchnikow of the Pasteur Institute showed that the cells, too, had an important role to play, not only by producing antibodies, but also by ingesting and destroying the invading bacteria.

In spite of the new knowledge of disease-producing organisms, the genesis of many epidemics and the mechanism of contagion remained mysterious until the demonstration of the part played by vectors, or intermediaries, in the transmission of contagion. The most notable of these transmitters was found to be the healthy human carrier, postulated by Pettenkofer for cholera as early as 1855. The role of the healthy human carrier was demonstrated by Loeffler, Roux, Yersin, Koch, Park, and others in the nineties. It was shown that healthy carriers were largely responsible for the spread of diphtheria, cholera, meningitis, typhoid fever, poliomyelitis, and dysentery. The second important step for the understanding of the genesis of infectious disease was the identification of animal carriers of parasitic organisms. It was already known that dogs carried rabies and certain worms, and it was realized that the fly very often transported infectious material from excrement to food. But in fact the transportation of infectious material by animals was usually far more complicated than the purely mechanical activities of the fly.

In most cases of animal transmission the disease-producing organism passes certain stages in the body of the animal, a phenomenon technically called metaxeny. This was demonstrated for the cestodes by Kuechenmeister in 1851. Leuckart and Melnikoff showed in 1868 that the dog louse carried the dog tapeworm in this way. In 1877 Sir Patrick Manson showed that the mosquito carried the *Filaria bancrofti*. Theobald Smith and Kilbourn in 1889 identified ticks as the carriers of the plasmodium of Texas cattle fever. David Bruce showed in 1894 that the tsetse fly was the carrier of the deadly trypanosoma of an African cattle disease. This set the stage for the immensely important discovery of Sir Ronald Ross in 1897 that the plasmodia of malaria, the most prevalent of all diseases, were carried by mosquitoes, identified as *Anopheles* by Grassi in 1898. In 1897 Simond and Ogata showed that fleas carried plague. In 1901 Walter Reed, Caroll, Lazear, and Agramonte of the U. S. Army, working on a hypothesis originated by the Cuban physician Juan Carlos Finlay, demonstrated that yellow fever was carried by the mosquito *Aedes aegypti,* the carrier of dengue. In 1909 Charles Nicolle showed that typhus was transmitted by lice, which also carry trench fever and relapsing fever. The discovery of carriers, even more than the isolation of disease-producing organisms, paved the way for more effective prevention of contagious diseases.

The consequences of the development of bacteriology were tremendous. It is impossible to overemphasize the importance of the fact that for the first time in history *causes* of numerous diseases became known. The way was opened for a replacement of symptomatic or empirical treatment by causal treatment and prevention. A definite answer could finally be given to the question as to whether the disease-producing agent was a "miasma," a chemical agent, or a living organism. The problem of the specificity of diseases was solved. The gap between the discoveries of pure science and their successful application in practice was bridged faster than ever before. This fact impressed the lay public with the potentialities of medicine more than any previous discovery. Rational treatment and prevention of infectious diseases became possible on an unprecedented scale. The whole of medicine was transformed, with the fields of public health and surgery undergoing a complete rejuvenation.

The function of the clinical concept of such diseases as tuberculosis and syphilis had been to unite a large number of clinical symptoms under one common denominator. These clinical concepts could now be confirmed. It is amazing how many disease units, originally isolated on purely clinical and pathological-anatomical grounds, were now identified and confirmed through bacteriological discovery. The value of clinical methods received a striking demonstration. Only a minority of disease units, such as Woodward's "typho-malarial" fever, were found to be imaginary.

Of course, the growth of bacteriology was not without its crises and disappointments. A great many bacteria that were isolated as producing cancer and other conditions were later found not to have the pathogenic qualities assigned to them in the first burst of enthusiasm. Many conditions, such as the pneumonias, appeared to be the result of something far more complex than the action of one single type of bacterium. And in their research on virus diseases the bacteriologists encountered technical obstacles which they could not master with their routine methods.

Eventually it became obvious that, though bacteria were a cause of many diseases, they were not the disease itself, as had often been thought in the first enthusiasm. Henle and Virchow had warned that there was a difference between disease cause and disease process, and their warning proved well founded. Bacteria were not the sole cause of disease. A great many more factors had to be considered beyond the mechanical encounter between a bacterium and a host. Constitutional, geographical, and social factors, which for decades had been completely neglected because of a blind trust in bacteriology, had to be reconsidered. It was realized that even knowledge of the parasitical cause of a disease, and of effective methods for its treatment, might still not bring about eradication of the disease if certain social and economic factors were unfavorable to full application of such knowledge. This is obvious in the case of malaria, tuberculosis, and syphilis. Medical knowledge is probably now sufficient to eradicate these diseases, but social conditions insure their continued existence.

In spite of these qualifications, in spite of the fact that in the total framework of science the rise of bacteriology was only one among the many great biological discoveries of the times, there is no doubt that from the strictly medical viewpoint it was the most important development of the eventful nineteenth century and perhaps of all recorded time.

Chapter 16

SURGERY AND GYNECOLOGY IN THE NINETEENTH CENTURY

Three factors were instrumental in the tremendous progress of surgery during the nineteenth century, quite apart from the abolition of the medieval distinction between medicine and surgery and the consequent social rehabilitation of the surgeon. These factors were localism, anesthesia, and asepsis. Each of them was an application of the insights of science to the field of surgery.

The influence of localism has been discussed in a previous chapter. The surgeon was necessarily "knife shy" as long as humoralism held sway. It was absurd for him to remove a tumor, for example, believing as he did that the tumor was only the expression of a dyscrasia; it was bound to grow again on the same or another spot. Localistic pathological anatomy, partially created by the surgeons and enthusiastically embraced by them, gave a new meaning to many operations. Surgical activity increased greatly decades before the invention of anesthesia and asepsis. A new type of surgeon arose, very different from the traditional type, whose main occupation had been the setting of fractures, treatment of wounds and venereal diseases, and amputation in case of war.

Despite his new knowledge and his new techniques, the surgeon still worked under two grave handicaps. The first of these handicaps was the almost inevitable wound infection as a result of which even "successful" operations more often than not ended in fatal septicemia. This infection was especially rampant in hospitals—called *seminaria mortis* by Leibnitz. It is easy to sympathize with the fear felt by former generations at the prospect of "going to the hospital." There the internal patient died from "hospital fever" (typhus), while the surgical patient mysteriously succumbed to "hospital gangrene." It was this latter difficulty that was solved by asepsis.

The history of modern asepsis begins on a tragic note and with a tragic figure. Almost a generation before the triumph of modern surgery, an obscure obstetrician discovered the clue to puerperal infection, which is identical with wound infection. He laid his gift at the feet of the medical world— and was laughed at, or at best ignored. This man, probably the finest product of the New Vienna School, was the Hungarian Ignaz P. Semmelweis (1818–1865), a personal friend of Rokitansky, Skoda, and Hebra.

While working at the first obstetric clinic of the University of Vienna, Semmelweis was struck by the marked difference between his and the second obstetric clinic in the number of puerperal mortalities. The first clinic's mortality rate was three times as high as the other's. Only the first clinic was open to medical students, while the second served for the instruction of midwives. Through a judicious analysis of autopsy reports, Semmelweis concluded in 1847 that puerperal fever in the first clinic was produced primarily by contact with the contaminated hands of doctors and medical students coming from the autopsy room. He demonstrated the truth of his conclusion by introducing the routine of handwashing with a chlorine solution before manual examination. The result was a dramatic reduction in puerperal mortality. Semmelweis not only uncovered the cause of puerperal fever but also realized its identity with wound fever. Few of his colleagues were impressed with his puerperal theory, and all of them ignored his contention that wound fever stemmed from the same cause. As a reward for his discovery he was dismissed from his position at the Vienna clinic and had to return to Budapest.

Semmelweis' discovery was by no means entirely original. Eighteenth-century British obstetricians like Alexander Gordon of Aberdeen and Charles White of Manchester had suspected that doctors carried the source of puerperal infection. However, they imagined the mechanism to be rather like the transfer of smallpox. They knew that cleanliness reduced puerperal mortality. Ideas almost identical with those of Semmelweis had been expressed by Oliver Wendell Holmes in 1843. But, meeting the same kind of malicious resistance which Semmelweis was to encounter, Holmes did not insist on his discovery; he limited himself to the teaching of anatomy and the fathering of poetry and a Supreme Court justice.

Semmelweis was original primarily in the unbending energy and zeal with which he championed the new principle. He saw the lives of thousands of mothers sacrificed every year in the hospitals through the ignorance of doctors. He preached, but he was not heard, and his mind became more and more obscured in his frantic fight against the stupid and costly conservatism of his colleagues. In 1865 Semmelweis died at the age of forty-seven from sepsis in an insane asylum in Vienna. When Joseph Lister heard in the 1880's of Semmelweis' work, he generously recognized that the credit for the introduction of the principle of asepsis into surgery belonged to Semmelweis.

The second great obstacle to large-scale surgery, in addition to wound infection and the resultant septicemia, was the inadequacy of the means available to surgeons for the control of pain. This restricted the scope of operations, intensified shock, and made speed essential. Future developments in surgery waited on the discovery of adequate pain-control methods.

Ether and nitrous oxide had served as sources of amusement at so-called "frolics" since the beginning of the century. European scientists, beginning with Sir Humphry Davy in 1800, had suggested the possibility of using such gases as anesthetics. But the decisive step in this direction was taken in the United States. In 1844 the Connecticut dentist Horace Wells (1815–1847) successfully started the practice of anesthetizing his patients with nitrous oxide. William Thomas

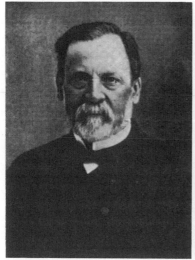 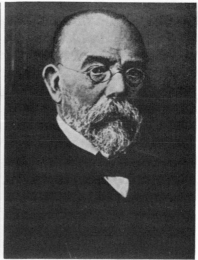

FIGURE 17. Louis Pasteur.   FIGURE 18. Robert Koch.

Green Morton (1819–1868), another dentist, was familiar with Wells's work. His preceptor, Dr. Charles T. Jackson (1805–1880) of Boston, drew his attention to sulfuric ether as a possible anesthetic. After successful use of ether in dental practice, Morton approached the famous Boston surgeon, John Collins Warren, and requested the trial of the new method in a surgical operation. The famous trial operation took place in Massachusetts General Hospital on October 16, 1846, and was a full success.

In spite of the unavoidable opposition of conservatives, the new method spread with great speed on both sides of the Atlantic. Its three promoters became embroiled in an ugly wrangle about priority. All died tragic deaths, Wells by suicide, Jackson insane, and Morton a pauper. The irony of fate is that none of them was in fact the first to practice gaseous anesthesia. Crawford W. Long (1815–1878) of Dansville, Georgia, had applied ether anesthesia as early as 1842. However, since he did not publish his discovery, it remained irrelevant to the introduction of anesthesia into medical practice.

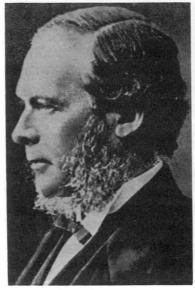 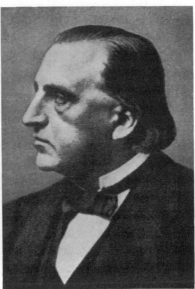

FIGURE 19. Lord Lister.   FIGURE 20. Jean Martin Charcot.

Sir James Young Simpson (1811–1870), professor of obstetrics in Edinburgh, had been one of the first to use ether in Europe. In 1847 he introduced the use of chloroform as an anesthetic. Chloroform became very popular and at times almost supplanted ether as the principal anesthetic agent. Since that time a great many other agents have been invented, techniques have been refined and improved, and anesthesia has become a specialty. The invention of general anesthesia was followed forty years later by the invention of various forms of local anesthesia. A local anesthetic, in the form of cocaine, was first applied in ophthalmology by Carl Koller in 1884. Conduction anesthesia was developed by W. S. Halsted in 1885, and infiltration anesthesia by C. L. Schleich in 1894. It seems unnecessary to elaborate on the extraordinary value of anesthesia and the great changes it brought about in all branches of surgery, including that of physiological experimentation.

Two decades after the introduction of anesthesia, the problem of wound infection was tackled again, this time by Joseph Lister (1827–1912). The last of the great Quaker physicians of the nineteenth century, Lister was shocked by the tremendous losses incurred in surgical practice. He was particularly struck by the difference in the mortality rate between cases of simple and complicated fracture. The main difference between simple and complicated factures is that the latter communicate with the air. The French chemist Louis Pasteur had just shown bacteria to be present everywhere in the air, and it occurred to Lister that bacteria from the air might enter the wound to produce the deadly septicemia. Lister thus began to apply Pasteur's discoveries by protecting open fractures against bacteria with carbolic acid, a disinfectant recommended by Jules Lemaire as early as 1860. Lister's results, which he started publishing in 1867, were astonishing. He soon extended the use of carbolic acid to all fields of surgery, calling his new principle the antiseptic principle. With Lister the days of "laudable pus" came to an end.

In spite of Lister's convincing results, acceptance of his new methods was neither rapid nor widespread. Only after the Germans (von Volkmann, Thiersch, Mikulicz, and others) had taken up his techniques in the early seventies did medical men in the United States, France, and eventually England, follow suit. Lister's clumsy methods were replaced in the 1880's by the technique of asepsis, chiefly developed by Schimmelbusch in von Bergmann's clinic in Berlin and by Octave Terrillon in Paris. In the classic Listerian procedure instruments, wound, and operator were all sprayed with carbolic acid. The new technique insured freedom from bacteria by the disinfection of the instruments with steam, the hands and the field of operation having been previously disinfected by means of various agents. Antisepsis and asepsis rejuvenated surgery entirely and transformed surgical wards, after centuries of hospital gangrene, into places which one could enter with the hope of leaving alive.

It should not be overlooked that a great number of smaller technical improvements and inventions contributed considerably to the rapid advance of surgery. The artery clamp was developed in 1862 by Koeberlé and Péan. Halsted improved the artery clamp and introduced the rubber glove. Carl Ruge described the biopsy with frozen sections in Berlin in 1878.

In the 1880's surgeons began to invade regions of the human body that they had never before dared to touch—the joints, the abdomen, the head, and the vertebral column. The leader in the first great period of abdominal surgery was the great Vienna surgeon, Theodor Billroth (1829–1894), the friend of Johannes Brahms. Billroth resected the oesophagus in 1872, the pylorus in 1881, and parts of the intestines in 1878. His pupil Woelfler introduced gastro-enterostomy in 1881. The period of appendectomy was opened by U. Kroenlein of Zurich in 1885 and in 1886 by Reginald Heber Fitz. Cholecystostomy was undertaken by J. M. Sims in 1878, and kidney removal by Gustav Simon in 1869. W. McEwey and Victor Horsley (1857–1916) started operating on tumors of the brain and of the spinal cord. Horsley was also active in gland surgery. This new surgical field, now opening for the first time, was primarily concerned with the removal of the thyroid gland in goiter or Graves' disease. Pioneers in this field were Theodor Kocher, J. L. Reverdin, and Anton Eiselsberg. Unfortunately, ignorance of the thyroid function and of the existence of the parathyroid glands led to the total removal of the gland in the early cases. The catastrophic consequences of this procedure were corrected speedily through the honest admission of failures by their authors.

Older operations, such as the removal of the cancerous breast and the reparation of hernias, were tremendously improved by William Stuart Halsted and Edoardo Bassini. Karl Thiersch introduced skin grafting. Outstanding English surgeons of the period were, in addition to Lister and Horsley, Sir James Paget, remembered through the two "Paget's diseases," the many-sided Sir William Macewen, and Sir Berkeley Moynihan, an abdominal surgeon. The United States, besides anesthesia, contributed the work of several outstanding gynecological surgeons, including Sims, Emmett, and the Atlee brothers. Their work, like that of the American dentists, was to be emulated in Europe. The Russians produced one outstanding surgeon in this period, Nikolai I. Pirogoff (1810–1881).

Obstetrics and gynecology are old surgical specialties. The same forces that rejuvenated surgery opened new horizons to them. The first ovariotomy was carried out with rare courage and understanding in the backwoods of Kentucky by Ephraim McDowell in 1809. McDowell was followed by John Light Atlee and Washington Lemuel Atlee in Pennsylvania. Ovariotomy became a routine operation in Europe following the work of two Englishmen, Thomas Spencer Wells, beginning in 1858, and Robert Lawson Tait in 1871. Tait also started to operate for tubal pregnancies and pyosalpinx, and he performed hysterectomies, an operation which was greatly improved by W. A. Freund in 1878. For centuries gynecological surgeons had been unable to deal effectively with the vesicovaginal fistula. Through experiments on female slaves James Marion Sims (1813–1883) of South Carolina developed the first reliable operation for this condition in 1852. Other Southern gynecological surgeons of this period were Thomas Addis Emmett and Robert Battey of Georgia. Cesarian section was established as a routine procedure through improvements introduced by Porro in 1876 and Saenger in 1882.

The contributions of Karl Siegmund Crédé (1819–1892) are not truly surgical in nature; yet they compare favorably with any new operative procedures of the period in terms of medical usefulness. Crédé introduced a method to express the placenta, which prevented much postnatal bleeding. And by the simple expedient of instilling an antiseptic silver nitrate solution into the eyes of every newborn, he did away with the infant gonorrheal eye infections which had been the cause of so much blindness.

Chapter 17

THE NEW SPECIALISM OF THE NINETEENTH CENTURY

The nineteenth century saw the development of the specialism which has become so characteristic of present-day medicine. The majority of the practicing doctors in the United States are now specialists, and sixty-six specialty boards have been formed. Specialism today does not call to mind the old broad divisions—medicine, surgery, obstetrics, and gynecology—which had existed for centuries; rather, it indicates the many independent subdivisions of surgery and medicine which came into being during the nineteenth century.

The diseases that formed the subject matter of these specialties had, of course, been studied before and had sometimes been dealt with separately in the literature. But the great increase in scientific knowledge during the nineteenth century for the first time made it possible, and even necessary, for medical men to limit their practice to the diseases of certain organs or organ groups. The invention of new instruments, such as the many "scopes," provided a further incentive for the formation of specialties. These instruments required special training for their proper use and often transformed completely the fields to which they were applied. It should also be remembered that localistic pathology favored the development of specialties. It is no accident that Vienna and Paris, and later Berlin, played such a large role in the history of specialties. Nonmedical factors exerted their influence, particularly the development of big cities and the multiplication of middle-sized cities able to furnish sufficient patients to allow specialization. There is little doubt that the public reacted very favorably to the idea of specialism, and that its growth and present magnitude are largely a result of public demand. The profession, represented by the general practitioner and general surgeon, strongly opposed the development of specialism, partly because specialism in the past had been associated with disreputable elements such as the traveling "stone-cutter" and the "oculist." The dangers inherent in specialization were also foreseen. Less noble reasons, including the traditional conservatism of the medical profession and the fear of losing patients, played their part in the widespread feelings against specialization.

The pattern of development was similar in all the specialties. Usually the budding specialists began by opening special dispensaries where they treated the poor without fee, thereby provoking less resistance from the profession. Once a specialty had been established, clinics were opened. Eventually chairs, societies, and specialist journals were founded.

It is convenient to divide the specialties for the purpose of this discussion into two groups, the surgical and the medical specialties. One of the earliest surgical specialties, orthopedics, was not primarily a product of the invention of new instruments, or even of those factors that influenced the general growth of surgery and its specialties, such as localism, anesthesia, and asepsis. Rather, its growth stemmed from the humanitarian interest in crippled children resulting from the Enlightenment. This is obvious in the work of Nicolas Andry (1658–1742), who coined the term "orthopedics" in 1741. In 1780 the first institute for deformed children was founded by J. A. Venel in Switzerland. Contemporaries of the great surgeons of the period of hospital medicine were orthopedic surgeons such as Delpech, Stromeyer, and Heine. They were still handicapped by the absence of asepsis and had to resort to subcutaneous operations. Valentine Mott failed to establish an orthopedic institute in New York City in 1840, but Heimann Berend succeeded in Berlin in 1851. University orthopedic clinics were opened everywhere between 1875 and

1900. Operative orthopedics developed parallel to the new surgery. Conservative methods also proved very successful, as in Adolf Lorenz' treatment of congenital hip dislocation.

Physiotherapy also owed its first reawakening, after a neglect of centuries, to the period of the Enlightenment. Massage and gymnastics, both closely related to orthopedics, received special attention. Rousseau, J. P. Frank, Tissot, and others were interested in these methods of physiotherapy. Their work was continued by the Frenchmen Desgenettes, Londe, and Amoros, and by the "Turners" in Germany. Gymnastics received a particularly strong impetus from the work of a Swedish layman, Per Henrik Ling, who started his medical gymnastics in 1813. Another Swede, Zander, introduced gymnastic apparatus in 1865. Intensive occupation with the Hippocratic writings on the part of Magne and Bonnet led to a revival of gymnastics in France in the fifties. The prevalent skeptical attitude in therapeutics toward drugs and bleeding contributed to the development of gymnastics. Experimental scientific work was started in the 1870's by Mosengeil, and such outstanding surgeons as Billroth, Langenbeck, and Bergmann took an intensive interest in gymnastics.

Ophthalmology remained to a large extent in the hands of quacks until the end of the eighteenth century. Jacques Daviel had considerably improved cataract operations in 1748. The Quaker Thomas Young (1783–1829), also outstanding as a physicist, engineer, and Egyptologist, cleared up a number of the problems of refraction. This made possible the first crystallization of the subject at the beginning of the nineteenth century. The first professor of ophthalmology was Joseph Baer in Vienna in 1812. John C. Saunders opened the first English eye infirmary in 1805, and the first eye infirmary in New York City was opened in 1820 in spite of the resistance of the profession. The field expanded tremendously with the invention of the ophthalmoscope by Helmholtz in 1851 and the fundamental work on refraction by F. C. Donders. The surgical aspects of the field progressed parallel with the general surgical renaissance, particularly

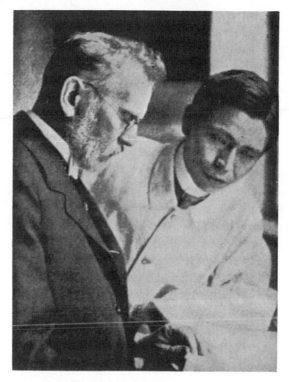

FIGURE 21. Paul Ehrlich and Hata.

under the leadership of Albrecht von Graefe (1828–1870), who introduced iridectomy and new operations for strabism and cataract. Consequently chairs of ophthalmology were founded in the sixties, and university clinics were opened in the seventies. The introduction of local anesthesia into ophthalmology by Koller in 1884 has already been mentioned.

In otology, which originally was combined with ophthalmology, the same stages of evolution can be observed: crystallization, enlargement through new diagnostic means, and surgical advance. Typical of the period of crystallization is the treatise of J. M. G. Itard (1773–1838), published in 1821. The perforated mirror was invented by Fr. Hofmann of Burgsteinfurt (1806–1886) in 1841, but it was really brought into general use by Adam Politzer (1835–1920) of Vienna.

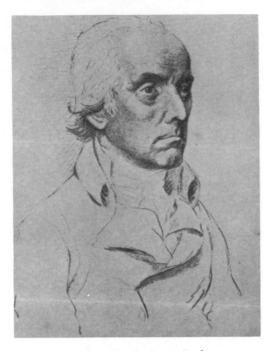

FIGURE 22. Benjamin Rush.

Surgical progress in otology is closely connected with the names of Sir William Robert Wilde (1815–1876) of Dublin—the father of the poet Oscar Wilde—and Hermann Schwartze (1847–1916) of Halle, who introduced the mastoid operation in the seventies. This operation has only recently lost its fundamental importance through the tremendous progress in chemotherapy. The first otology chairs in Germany were founded in the sixties.

Rhinology and laryngology developed comparatively late. They became independent specialties only when they were combined with otology, after this discipline, in turn, had been separated from ophthalmology. The technical invention basic to this development was indirect laryngoscopy. Many efforts at laryngoscopy had been made before, but the problem was first solved by a layman, the Spanish singer Manuel

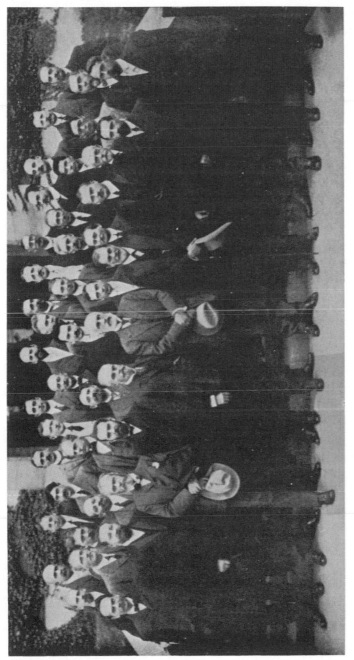

FIGURE 23. Sigmund Freud at Clark University, 1909.

First row, left to right: Franz Boas, E. B. Tichener, William James, William Stern, Leo Burgerstein, G. Stanley Hall, Sigmund Freud, Carl G. Jung, Adolf Meyer, H. S. Jennings. *Second row*: C. E. Seashore, Joseph Jastrow, J. McK. Cattell, E. F. Buchner, E. Katzenellenbogen, Ernest Jones, A. A. Brill, William H. Burnham, A. F. Chamberlain. *Third row*: Albert Schinz, J. A. Magni, B. T. Baldwin, F. Lyman Wells, G. M. Forbes, E. A. Kirkpatrick, Sandor Ferenczi, E. C. Sanford, J. P. Porter, Sakyo Kanda, Hikoso Kakise. *Fourth row*: G. E. Dawson, S. P. Hayes, E. B. Holt, C. S. Berry, G. M. Whipple, Frank Drew, J. W. A. Young, L. N. Wilson, K. J. Karlson, H. H. Goddard, H. I. Klopp, S. C. Fuller.

García, in 1854. Tuerck and Czermak of Vienna also achieved solutions in 1857 and 1858 respectively. In 1873 a laryngological society was founded in New York. The invention of local anesthesia was of great importance for the development in the eighties of operative rhinology for operations on the nasal septum and the sinuses. Bronchoscopy was introduced by Gustav Killian of Mainz in 1898 and developed by Chevalier Jackson of Philadelphia in 1900.

The history of otorhinolaryngology provides excellent examples of the fact that the boundaries between the different specialties are fluid. New combinations occur at all times. Originally combined with ophthalmology, otology was later joined with rhinology and laryngology. And bronchoscopy, at first an important part of laryngology, is now claimed by other specialties such as chest surgery. The basic instrument for the development of urology was the lithopropter, introduced in Paris in 1824. The next important acquisition, the cystoscope, was invented by Max Nitze of Vienna in 1876.

The development of the medical specialties paralleled that in surgery. Pediatrics, like orthopedics, gained strength from the philosophy of the Enlightenment. The French philosopher Rousseau had energetically expounded the merits of healthful child rearing. The books of the Swede Nils von Rosenstein (1752), of George Armstrong (1767), and of William Cadogan (1748) are typical of the Enlightenment pediatrics. Being itself the application of internal medicine to a certain age group, pediatrics followed closely in its own development the developmental stages of internal medicine. Hospital medicine was represented by the Frenchman Charles Billard (1800–1832), who published his fundamental treatise in 1828, four years before his premature death from tuberculosis. This makes him a kind of Laennec of pediatrics. The classic treatise on pediatrics in the second half of the nineteenth century was written entirely in the spirit of Paris hospital medicine by F. Rilliet and A. Barthez (1843). The British representative of hospital medicine in pediatrics was Charles West (1818–1891). The statistical studies of the

Belgian Adolphe Quetelet (1796–1874) did much to illuminate for medicine the biological peculiarities of the child. The first children's hospitals were opened in Paris in 1802 and in London in 1852.

Laboratory medicine found its expression in pediatrics during the second half of the nineteenth century in the chemical analysis of foodstuffs and in metabolic studies. At that time it was of particular importance to study the respective composition of cow's milk and human milk. This was accomplished by Franz Simon in 1848 and by Philipp Biedert in 1869. Bacteriology influenced pediatrics no less than general medicine, and the progress in histology led to a better understanding of the hematology of childhood. Outstanding pediatricians of this period include Camerer, Feer, Escherich, Finkelstein, Czerny, Heubner, and Rotch, who were all primarily concerned with the problems of infant feeding.

Dermatology crystallized in the eighteenth century, as is reflected by Lorry's pioneer treatise of 1777. Jean Louis Alibert (1768–1837) was the real founder of the discipline, although his system—he was strongly under the systematizing influence of the eighteenth century—was soon superseded by the more modern approach of the English Quaker Robert Willan (1757–1812). Ferdinand von Hebra (1816–1880) of Vienna, the founder of a great school, introduced the histological or pathological approach. The important repercussions of bacteriology on dermatology are represented by the work of Raymond Sabouraud (1864–1938) and Paul Unna (1850–1929). Dermatology as an independent specialty was established in the 1870's.

Dermatology had been traditionally combined with syphilology and the study of venereal diseases in general. Probably the two greatest syphilologists of the century were the Baltimore-born Frenchman, Philippe Ricord (1799–1889), and Jean-Alfred Fournier (1832–1914). Ricord definitely established the independent existence of gonorrhea and syphilis and laid down the division of syphilis into its three stages. Fournier's work covered the whole field of syphilis, but he is particularly remembered for establishing statistically the connection between syphilis and tabes (locomotor ataxia). His work in this field was almost simultaneous with that of the German neurologist Erb. Sir Jonathan Hutchinson (1828–1913) is remembered for his work in heredosyphilis. The discovery of the causative organisms of venereal disease by Neisser, Ducrey, and Schaudinn was followed by important progress in diagnostics and treatment in the twentieth century. The far-reaching recession of syphilis during the last forty years has changed considerably the physiognomy of the specialty dermatology-venerology, as well as that of psychiatry and neurology. The latter disciplines were also strongly influenced by the rise of neurosurgery.

Neurology had been practiced for a long time within the limits of internal medicine. It developed relatively late as an independent discipline because of the late development of the underlying neuro-anatomy and physiology. The fact that neurology was still largely virgin soil in the nineteenth century made it an attractive field to a number of outstanding clinicians. Perhaps another explanation of its attractiveness to clinicians was the fact that, despite its reliance upon the laboratory, it preserved more aspects of the old hospital medicine than any of the other subdivisions of internal medicine. The German neurological school, which in the course of the century produced men like Friedreich, Erb, Leyden, Nothnagel, Oppenheim, Quincke, and Struempell, was fathered by Moritz Romberg. It was Romberg who in 1846 described the sign for locomotor ataxia in the first formal treatise on nervous diseases. Guillaume Benjamin Duchenne (1806–1875) was the pioneer of French nineteenth-century neurology. He used electrodiagnosis and electrotherapeutics extensively. He described bulbar paralysis, explained poliomyelitis as due to lesions of the anterior horns, and assigned the cause of locomotor ataxia to lesions of the posterior columns of the spinal cord. Driven by an indomitable urge for research, he haunted the wards of Paris hospitals for forty years. Shy and a poor speaker, he never held an official position, and his genius was recognized by few during his lifetime.

Jean Martin Charcot (1825–1893), who was originally a pathologist and remained a general clinician all his life, was induced to concentrate his interest on neurology when, in 1862, he became physician to the great hospital of the Salpetrière, which harbored an enormous amount of neurological material. There he founded his famous clinic, to which students flocked from the four corners of the earth. Charcot, who maintained the primacy of clinical observation throughout his life, is probably the most representative clinician of the period. As a neurologist he is best known for his work on locomotor ataxia (its gastric crises and the joint affection named after him), hysteria, and muscular atrophy. The great tradition of French neurology was carried on by Charcot's pupils, Pierre Marie (1853–1940), Jules Déjerine (1849–1917), and Joseph Babinski (1857–1932). Marie described acromegaly and connected it with pituitary pathology. Babinski is particularly remembered for his studies on the reflexes and for his new concept of hysteria, which superseded that of his teacher Charcot.

Most representative of the English neurologists was John Hughlings Jackson (1834–1911). He was known for his studies of aphasia and of convulsions following cortex lesion (Jacksonian epilepsy). He did much to establish the use of the ophthalmoscope in the diagnosis of neurological disease. He played an important part in establishing the notion of the "levels of integration" in the central nervous system, an idea conceived under the influence of evolutionary theories in general biology. The outstanding American neurologist of the period was Silas Weir Mitchell (1829–1914) of Philadelphia, whose rest cure was accepted internationally. Mitchell was also a successful poet and novelist. George Miller Beard (1839–1883) of New York introduced the concept of neurasthenia in 1869.

Psychiatry is combined with neurology under one specialty board. This arrangement is quite logical, since mental disease is probably ultimately a disease of the brain, and thus one of the diseases of the nervous system. In fact, in the cases of general paresis and senile dementia, typical pathological changes in the brain can be demonstrated. Yet for the most important and widespread mental diseases, such as schizophrenia, paranoia, and manic-depressive states, no anatomical or physiological basis has been found, and no knowledge of causes exists comparable to that achieved in other branches of medicine. This remains true in spite of extensive research during more than a century. Psychiatry is therefore forced to operate on a different level from the rest of medicine, and its accomplishments often fall short, through no fault of its adepts, of those of other branches. Its scope, on the other hand, is immeasurably greater than that of any other specialty. Quite apart from the mental diseases as such, there is an element of mental disturbance in practically every disease.

The comparatively undeveloped state of psychiatry is easy to understand in the light of the fact that psychiatry is by far the youngest of the great branches of medicine. Psychiatry could develop only after the Enlightenment had put mental disease back into the hands of medical men, and after insane asylums had slowly been transformed from a mixture of zoo and penitentiary into mental hospitals. Only then could psychoses be studied seriously. Neuroses had fared somewhat better, since they were "ambulatory diseases." They had received the attention of such practitioners as Sydenham, Cheyne, and Trotter. Because of its late development psychiatry carried into the nineteenth century some of the traits of earlier periods of medicine, such as the preoccupation with prognosis, classification, and speculative systems, so characteristic of eighteenth-century medicine.

Mention has already been made of Pinel, whose pioneer psychiatric treatise was published in 1801 and who introduced humane practices into asylums in 1794. An institution for the insane, based on similar humane principles, was founded by the English Quaker William Tuke at York in 1796.

Pinel was followed by a whole group of French psychiatrists, headed by his pupil Jean Étienne Dominique Esquirol (1772–1840). Esquirol's greatness stems from his non-dogmatic attitude. His primary concern was clinical observation, not classification of mental disease or interpretation of it exclusively in terms of either somatic or psychological causation. He saw that masturbation and other so-called "causes" of insanity were in fact only symptoms. Recognizing that the rationalists of the Enlightenment were too much concerned with the intellectual aspects of mental disease, he held that its roots were primarily emotional and affective— or "moral," to use the vocabulary of the time. His treatment, too, was nondogmatic. Esquirol did much for the improvement of mental institutions and was an early exponent of statistics and public health.

Other accomplishments of the French school include Antoine Laurent Bayle's discovery of general paresis in 1822. This disease was at this time extremely prevalent. Esquirol claimed that 50 per cent of his inmates were paretics. Falret and Baillarger described circular insanity in 1853. Georget emphasized the role of the brain in mental disease as early as 1820. Noteworthy among the English psychiatrists of the period were John Conolly (1794–1860), protagonist of the no-restraint system, and J. C. Pritchard (1786–1848), who coined the notion of moral insanity in his treatise of 1835.

With the work of Wilhelm Griesinger (1817–1868) leadership in psychiatry passed into the hands of Germans. Griesinger had already distinguished himself by excellent work with infectious diseases, including his discovery of hookworm anemia and in his promotion of a new physiological, antiromantic medicine in Germany. German psychiatry had spent its forces in the early nineteenth century in fruitless battles between the "somaticists" and the "psychologists." Nasse and Jacobi can be taken as representatives of the former, and Heinroth and Ideler of the latter. Griesinger attempted a synthesis, developing such modern-sounding psychological notions as ego structure, wish fulfillment through symptoms, and frustration. His approach was dynamic, not purely symptomatological. Yet his bias, and that of the German school after him, remained somatic. Griesinger was also a practical reformer, sponsoring agricultural colonies and family care.

Somaticism found new support in the degeneration theories of Bénédict Morel (1809–1873) and Jacques Moreau de Tours (1804–1884), popularized later by Cesare Lombroso (1836–1909). It seemed easier to find so-called stigmata than to discover relevant brain lesions. The vogue of Darwinism reinforced these hereditary-constitutional and basically fatalistic ideas.

The present-day classification of mental disease is due to Emil Kraepelin (1856–1927). Kraepelin attempted to develop psychiatry along the lines of the neurophysiological psychology of Wundt. His excellent laboratory studies on fatigue and the psychic effect of alcoholism actually had little bearing on his main work. His contributions were rooted in clinical observation. Following Kahlbaum he no longer made single symptoms (excitement, depression, and so on) the basis of his analysis, but rather the total picture of the disease over time. His threefold classification—dementia praecox, paranoia, manic-depressive psychosis—seems more practical and closer to reality than any of the preceding classifications, but it was still purely symptomatic. Little psychotherapy and psychology can be found in Kraepelin's work.

His orientation was further developed in this respect by Eugen Bleuler (1857–1939), who also replaced the notion of dementia precox with that of schizophrenia. Ernst Kretschmer's *Constitution and Character* (1921), which connects certain types of body build and certain types of character with certain psychoses, has been equally suggestive for constitutional and for psychiatric studies.

By the end of the nineteenth century psychiatry had come to a dead end. The dominant somaticism had not given a satisfactory explanation of most mental diseases, nor had it provided effective methods of treatment. Occupational therapy was initiated by Ferrus, and rather generally used in the 1870's. But what little treatment existed was empirical, haphazard, and symptomatic. Even the more successful somatic treatments of the present day suffer from the same shortcomings.

Against this background of therapeutic despair and intellectual frustration it is easy to understand the tremendous influence that psychoanalysis, the doctrine of Sigmund Freud and his followers, acquired in modern psychiatry. Freud was originally a neurophysiologist and always believed in the organic cause of mental disease. But he had the daring to renounce temporarily vain somaticist efforts and to operate on the only accessible level, the psychological one. He tried to understand the dynamics of mental disease in psychological terms. In a situation where so pitifully little could be done, it was but natural that many would embrace a system to which practical successes and a progressive character could be ascribed, problematical as many of its theoretical foundations might be from a scientific point of view. Psychoanalysis, like earlier methods of psychotherapy, was of little avail when confronted with psychoses such as schizophrenia and manic-depressive insanity; but it has been very beneficial in the treatment of neuroses like hysteria and compulsion neurosis.

Psychoanalysts themselves trace modern psychotherapy back to F. Anton Mesmer (1734–1815), who was stigmatized as a quack by his contemporaries. Mesmer thought that he had discovered a specific magnetic force in humans and that this force could be transferred through the laying on of hands. He proved extremely successful in his practice based on this system. Mesmer was fundamentally neither a quack nor a mystic; he was a typical rationalist and speculative systematist in the eighteenth-century tradition. His misfortune was that he was born too late, when the period of systems had gone and when enough was known about magnetism to disprove his claims. Like many other therapists of all times, he was unable to see that his successes were due, not to his non-existent magnetic force, but to powerful suggestion. Mesmer himself probably did not practice hypnotism. It was developed by his pupils like Puységur.

Mesmerism found a courageous and enthusiastic defender in England in the person of John Elliotson (1791–1868). Scientific hypnotism could develop only when the results of mesmerism were accepted but its underlying theory discarded. This was the accomplishment of James Braid (1795–1861) of Manchester, who in 1843 published his *Neurypnology, or the Rationale of Nervous Sleep*. Independently of mesmerism, British surgeons had become acquainted with hypnotism in India. Esdaile's use of hypnotism in surgery has already been discussed. In France, Liébault and Bernheim developed the systematic psychotherapeutic use of suggestion, while the school of the Salpetrière, under Charcot, preferred to use hypnosis.

It was in Paris and Nancy that the young Austrian neurologist Sigmund Freud (1856–1939) studied these new psychotherapeutic methods. After his return to Vienna he began to work on new techniques in cooperation with Joseph Breuer, who had begun similar work in 1881. Their contribution, later to be called psychoanalysis, was submitted to the public for the first time in 1893 in their book on hysteria. Their technique, as reported in this work, was to have the patient report under hypnosis former traumatic and repressed psychological experiences. This technique was named "catharsis." This method had already been used in 1889 by Charcot's pupil, Pierre Janet. Freud subsequently discarded hypnosis, parted from Breuer, and developed his own elaborate theoretical system, which makes repression of sexual urges the central theme of psychology and psychopathology. Thanks to Freud's courage, intelligence, and ability as a writer and sect organizer, his system spread all over the world. Elements of his technique and doctrine have been adopted even by those who feel that in the successes of orthodox psychoanalysts the prominent factors are often, not the "rationalizations" of patient and physician, but the age-old mechanisms of confession and suggestion. Of Freud's many pupils mention can be made only of Carl Gustav Jung (born 1875) and Alfred Adler (1870–1937), who developed their own systems of depth psychology. Adler's "inferiority complex" has served as a valuable explanatory concept. Psychiatry is still rather helpless when dealing with drug addiction. A grandiose attempt at prevention and reform, the American prohibition of alcohol (1920–1933), was an utter failure.

In connection with the rise of specialties, the origins of the modern nursing profession cannot be neglected. Up to the middle of the nineteenth century nursing was in the hands either of nuns or of uneducated helpers of low quality. The first school for nurses was opened in 1836 by the German clergyman Theodor Fliedner in Kaiserswerth on the Rhine. The Fliedner institution served as inspiration to Florence Nightingale (1823–1910), an English lady from the upper strata of society, endowed with an indomitable energy and great ability. Her spectacular accomplishments in the abominable field hospitals of the Crimean War gave her the authority and the power to rejuvenate nursing in the English-speaking countries. She opened a school for nurses at St. Thomas' Hospital in 1860. The first training school for nurses in the United States was opened in 1873 by Elizabeth Blackwell (1821–1910), who was also the first woman M.D. in this country (1849). In the twentieth century, nursing in turn has been subdivided into several branches, and other auxiliary medical specialists have arisen, such as the laboratory technician, the x-ray technician, and the medical social worker. All these innovations have greatly improved medical care, but they have also made it more and more expensive, primarily because treatment occurs increasingly in hospitals, with their ever-more costly technological equipment.

Chapter 18

PUBLIC HEALTH AND PROFESSIONAL DEVELOPMENTS IN THE NINETEENTH CENTURY

Sir William Osler once called the modern period the age of preventive medicine. The truth of this statement is obvious once it is realized that the great accomplishment of modern medicine—the dramatically increased life expectancy in Western countries from forty years in 1850 to seventy years in 1950—is due much more to preventive than to curative medicine. Miraculous and admirable as the new antibiotics, for instance, may be, they have never saved nearly as many lives as the rather prosaic procedure of pasteurizing milk. Oliver Wendell Holmes was an early proponent of this view when he said, "The bills of mortality are more affected by drainage than this or that method of medical practice." The mundane character of preventive medicine has made it a stepchild in the eyes of medical history and in the sympathies of the larger public. Even in this book, the history of preventive medicine has played second fiddle to the history of clinical medicine. Only very recently the underestimation of preventive medicine has been replaced, at least in some places, and often under political influences, by an equally irrational belief in its unlimited powers.

Both individual hygiene and public hygiene owe an enormous debt to bacteriology. But this should not obscure the fact that preventive medicine, although sometimes hard to recognize through its religious or philosophical trimmings, is as old as human societies. We have encountered it among primitives, in Egypt, in Babylonia, among the ancient Jews, in Rome, and in the Middle Ages. We have observed the great preventive medicine movement of the eighteenth century, the fruit of the philosophical Enlightenment. We have seen that this movement was much rather the consequence of the will and the necessity to do something about public health than the result of new scientific insight. And we have seen that this approach achieved results and led to new discoveries. The same approach characterizes the first of the preventive medicine movements of the nineteenth century, the sanitary movement.

The sanitary movement was well under way before the great discoveries of bacteriology. It received its stimulus from the utilitarian philosophy of such thinkers as Jeremy Bentham, and it grew out of the needs of the new industrial society. Plague, leprosy, scurvy, and smallpox had receded from Western and Central Europe before their true nature was known. But the health situation was still appalling. Malaria prevailed in the country slums; typhus, typhoid fever, and tuberculosis were rife in the slums of the cities. A particularly strong incentive to the development of preventive medicine was given by the four great cholera pandemics which after 1830 swept Europe and the whole world, sparing neither rich nor poor. Cholera was once called by Robert Koch "our best ally" in the fight for better hygiene. Its dramatic effects frightened legislators into taking progressive measures far more rapidly than the creeping death resulting from tuberculosis or typhoid.

Unhygienic conditions in factories were the more appalling because of the widespread use of child labor. In the big cities the death rate had reached such levels by the middle of the nineteenth century that there were serious doubts whether sufficient hands would be available for the factories, and whether enough able-bodied recruits could be found for the general draft armies of the Continent. The big-city slums represented reservoirs of infectious diseases and epidemics, menacing not only the poor, but the life and health of the upper classes as well.

In England and Germany the hygiene movement of the Enlightenment seems to have experienced a decline at the end of the eighteenth and the beginning of the nineteenth century. But it was vigorously promoted in France. In fact, France assumed the lead in hygiene at this time, as it had done in most other branches of medicine. The work of French hygienists, particularly of René Louis Villermé (1782–1863), was an inspiration to German, British, and American authors. This French movement was overshadowed by the large-scale practical achievements in England after the passage of the General Health Act of 1848.

The driving spirit of the new English sanitary movement was, typically enough, an outsider, the lawyer Edwin Chadwick (1800–1890). He was a pupil and former secretary of Jeremy Bentham, the philosopher who strove for the greatest good for the greatest number. Chadwick's 1842 report on the health of the laboring classes revealed an ugly and dangerous situation. Chadwick had a counterpart in the United States in the person of a Boston merchant, Lemuel Shattuck (1793–1859), who made an equally famous report to the Massachusetts Sanitary Commission in 1850. Chadwick's closest collaborator was Dr. Southwood Smith (1816–1904), another pupil of Jeremy Bentham. Chadwick's statistical evidence was based to a large extent on the outstanding statistical work of Dr. William Farr (1807–1883), who in 1839 entered the Registrar General's office and started publishing his classic letters on the causes of death in England. Of the other outstanding English public health men of the period, Sir John Simon (1816–1904) was perhaps most influential. He was the first health officer of London, and later was medical officer to the General Board of Health. Although the General Board of Health operated on the erroneous "filth" theory of disease, its successes were striking. According to the filth theory, miasmatic hazes rising from decaying matter, rather than contagion and micro-organisms, were supposed to cause epidemics. But cleaning filth from the slums helped, whatever the underlying theory.

A much deeper understanding of the spread of infectious diseases was contributed by the English epidemiologists John Snow (1813–1858), also an outstanding anesthetist, and William Budd (1811–1880). Snow showed in 1849 that cholera was a water-borne disease, and in 1854 he proved his point conclusively in his classic treatise on the Broad Street pump. Budd demonstrated in 1856 that typhoid was also water-borne. Another milestone in epidemiology was Peter Panum's study of measles in the Faroe Islands in 1845.

A strong hygiene movement arose at about this time in Germany under the leadership of Max von Pettenkofer (1818–1901). Pettenkofer, father of the ground-water level theory, operated under erroneous assumptions with regard to contagion and was unsympathetic to bacteriology—to the extent of swallowing a virulent cholera culture in 1892 without evil effects (An earlier, mild attack had probably made him immune). But his practical achievements were considerable.

He made Munich a healthy city, as Virchow had done for Berlin. Pettenkofer went beyond the application of such ordinary measures as the improvement of water supply and sewage disposal; a trained physiologist and chemist, he was the first to submit all aspects of hygiene to experimental analysis, systematically investigating the effects of such factors as food, clothing, and housing. He was thus the father of modern scientific hygiene. He occupied the first chair of experimental hygiene in Munich in 1865.

The prebacteriological hygienists fought against "filth and stench." While this was insufficient, it went far toward eliminating many disease causes and disease carriers such as rats and lice. The prebacteriological hygiene movement concentrated on the fight against overcrowded housing, polluted water supplies, bad sewage, adulterated food, and child labor. It fought for isolation of those suffering from infectious diseases. It urged control of dangerous trades involving occupational intoxications from contact with lead or phosphorus. Under the leadership of Virchow and Hermann Cohn, school hygiene was vigorously developed. Better sewers and water supplies appeared in Western Europe after 1850. Pure food laws were introduced in the 1870's. Chairs of hygiene had been founded in the sixties.

Bacteriology led to unprecedented advances in preventive medicine. Direct attack against certain diseases could now replace haphazard measures. The incidence of typhoid fever and diphtheria could be rapidly reduced through control of the water and milk supplies, through control of carriers, and through immunization. After the identification of the mosquito as the carrier of yellow fever, William Crawford Gorgas (1854–1919) was able to carry out his spectacularly successful campaigns against yellow fever in Cuba and Panama, which won him world fame. Parallel discoveries made possible the effective control of malaria. The first great campaigns against malaria were directed by Sir Ronald Ross, the discoverer of the transmission of malaria by mosquitos. Gorgas, too, played his part in malaria control. As a whole the fight against water-borne diseases has been more successful than that against air-borne diseases.

Preventive medicine did not confine itself to the field of infectious diseases. The appearance of handbooks for occupational hygiene by Hirt, Layet, and Eulenburg in 1871 and 1876 illustrate the intense interest in the field in Europe. In the attack on occupational diseases outstanding work was done in the United States by Alice Hamilton. Child mortality was considerably reduced by the spread of better nutritional methods. The first campaign against goiter, through mass consumption of iodine in regions of iodine-deficient water supplies, was undertaken in this country by Marine in 1917. The introduction of state health insurance in Germany in 1884 proved to be a valuable preventive measure.

Preventive medicine did not rely entirely on legal methods of enforcement; educational methods received increasing attention. Through them, hygienic standards have changed completely. A hundred years ago one took a bath only when sick. The United States pioneered in one special field of preventive medicine, that of mental hygiene. Mental hygiene had long been promoted by doctors in individual cases, but mass application started only with the founding of the mental hygiene movement in New York in 1909.

The public health movement has produced a new type of doctor, the nontreating doctor. For the first time in history large numbers of medical men no longer treat individuals but deal exclusively with the health of larger groups of people. Another type of nontreating doctor is the nonpracticing scientist whose role has become more and more important since the middle of the last century. As professorships and Nobel prizes show, this role can even be played by nonmedical men and women.

The appearance of the nontreating doctor is only one of the many changes experienced by the medical profession during the nineteenth century under the influence of new scientific developments. Old problems, such as the separation of medicine and surgery, had disappeared. Through "academization" the barber-surgeons had become doctors, just as the toothpullers had become dentists, the spicers pharmacists, and the blacksmiths veterinarians. Scientific progress had solved the problem of decline in social standing that the profession had felt so painfully in the 1840's. But scientific progress also created new problems. Medical care has now become incomparably more effective than it was a hundred or even fifty years ago, but it has also become incomparably more expensive. In 1870 an office call cost twenty-five cents, a house call fifty to seventy-five cents. The large investment in education, especially specialist education, and the high cost of apparatus force the modern doctor to charge much higher fees than his grandfather did. The cost of medical care may partially explain certain negative aspects of the health situation of the American people today. In the Second World War, for instance, 40 per cent of the twenty-two million young men examined for the draft were rejected. Medical care is financially out of reach of many families at a time when demand for it is continually increasing. It is this combination of circumstances that has led to the pressure for governmental action, and the general tendency toward the welfare state.

Already the state has everywhere taken over the care of tuberculosis and mental disease, whose chronic character makes the cost of treatment prohibitive for the overwhelming majority of the population. Russia adopted some state controls over medicine as early as 1864 and since the revolution of 1917 has been operating exclusively with civil service physicians and *feldschers*. Germany started an obligatory health insurance system in 1884, and similar systems have been gradually adopted by all European countries. The British system was greatly extended after the Second World War. The state insurance systems have produced not only problems with simulation but also general ethical and loyalty conflicts for the doctors. In the United States the relatively high incomes of the major part of the population and the fear that an obligatory health insurance might be misused for political purposes have been factors in avoiding major reforms. So far the efforts to meet the difficulties of the new situation in this country have been restricted, up to the Medicare laws of 1965, to voluntary schemes. Hospital insurance and voluntary sickness insurance are good examples. The United States has pioneered in one particular attempt to adapt medical practice to new conditions by the formation of group practices. The best known became the Mayo Clinic of Rochester, Minnesota. Since the 1860's (Zurich, 1864; Paris, 1868), women have been admitted to medical schools. They have made increasing use of these opportunities, and by so doing, they have changed the face of medicine.

In the Middle Ages the priestly character of the physician gave him financial security. His secularization in modern times has made him once more a kind of shopkeeper, competing on the open market. Problems arising from competition among doctors were not quite so urgent as long as doctors were scarce and dealt mainly with a small number of wealthy patients. The masses were left to the barber-surgeons. But with the rise of industrial capitalism the number of doctors and prospective patients increased, while the relative number of wealthy few declined. Competition among doctors, and between doctors and quacks, grew to be a plague to the profession, and educational standards tended to deteriorate.

Attempts to control competition among doctors through codes of ethics date from the eighteenth century; Percival's code is an example. But in the nineteenth century these attempts acquired a more systematic character. It was realized that only through large-scale professional organization could the medical profession keep its professional competition within reasonable limits and elevate professional standards to such heights that the help of the state against quackery could justifiably be invoked. This was the task achieved by the large professional organizations founded around the middle of the nineteenth century—the British Medical Association in 1832, the American Medical Association in 1847, and the German Aerzteverein in 1872. There are, of course, no such unionlike structures in socialist countries. In the Soviet Union 75 per cent of the doctors are women, and there are almost as many *feldschers* as there are medical specialists.

Chapter 19

MEDICINE IN THE UNITED STATES
PRIOR TO 1900

In so far as medical events in the United States have had a bearing on international medicine, they have been dealt with in the previous pages. Such events are not too frequent in the short history of our country. It is rather surprising that there are so many of them in that historically short period of time. To those who live and work in the United States the history of medicine in this country has an additional significance. Their daily medical experiences are often the result of specific national traditions as well as more general historical trends. It is thus desirable to give here a short survey of the broad lines of the development of medicine in the United States up to 1900.

The United States was a new country; yet its roots were firmly grounded in an older civilization. It was faced with the problem of assimilating as rapidly as possible the attainments of the mother-countries of Europe. Consequently the problem of education and educational standards—of the adequate transmission of the best existing knowledge—was of prime importance in the formative period of United States medicine.

In the early Colonial period there were hardly any physicians and only a few surgeons. Health conditions were horrible, with one-half of the Mayflower's passengers dying within three months of their arrival. But the supply of doctors has so far always depended on the wealth of a society rather than on its health conditions. As a rule the only educated men in the struggling young colonies were the clergy, as had been true in medieval Europe and in the early stages of civilization in many parts of the world. It is therefore not surprising that the practice of medicine was largely carried on by the clergy. One Samuel Fuller, for instance, who came over on the Mayflower, was equally active in medical and in theological affairs. His wife functioned as a midwife. It is no accident, either, that the first American medical publication, a broadside on smallpox published in Boston in 1677, was written by a physician-clergyman, Thomas Thatcher. Cotton Mather, the well-known witch-hunting clergyman, has to his credit a rather enlightened and courageous attitude in the medical field. He had read in the *Transactions* of the Royal Society about the new inoculation method, and he persuaded a Boston practitioner, Zabdiel Boylston, to apply it in the 1721 epidemic. Poor Boylston became the object of much abuse as a reward for his courageous innovation.

By the end of the Colonial and the beginning of the National period the new country had reached a considerable level of civilization, of material and cultural wealth. This progress is reflected in the medical field, particularly in the high achievements of medicine in Philadelphia. American culture contributed such figures as Benjamin Franklin and Thomas Jefferson to the international movement of the Enlightenment. Benjamin Thompson and William Charles Wells, both Royalist refugees, became luminaries of European science. The first hospital in the United States proper—not in this hemisphere; hospitals in the French and Spanish colonies came much earlier—was founded in Philadelphia in 1752 under the inspiration of Benjamin Franklin. In 1765 the first medical school in the United States was opened, again in Philadelphia. The only means of training physicians up to this time had been the preceptorial system under which the future doctor was apprenticed to an older man for from four to seven years. This was a reversion to the archaic form of medical education observed in ancient Greece and India. Only a very few of these preceptor-trained doctors were able to augment this training by postgraduate studies in Europe. It has been estimated that in 1775 there were thirty-five hundred physicians in this country, of which number only four hundred held a university medical degree. There is no breakdown between physicians and surgeons in this figure, as there would have been in any corresponding European survey, because the vicious separation between physician and surgeon never took root in this country. The hard beginnings did not allow such European niceties, and after conditions had improved the separation fortunately was never introduced. This is undoubtedly one of the reasons for the early excellence of American surgery. In the late eighteenth century legal regulation of medical practice began to be established in states like New York and New Jersey, unfortunately to be abandoned in the explosive expansion of the nineteenth century. Under prevailing conditions the preceptorial system was by no means a poor system of education. The profession included a great many competent men who made excellent tutors. As a whole the general level of medical education was probably higher at the end of the eighteenth century than it was around the middle of the nineteenth century.

Such Americans as could afford a foreign education at the time usually turned to Edinburgh, then one of the world centers of medicine. American students usually showed very good judgment in the choice of European schools, and their predilection is in general an excellent indication of the leading medical centers of the time. This can be called the "Edinburgh period" in the history of American medicine, and later a "Paris" and a "German" period can be distinguished. John Morgan (1735–1789), founder of the Philadelphia Medical School and for a time Surgeon General of Washington's armies, was a graduate of Edinburgh. So were other outstanding Philadelphia men of the early period, including the obstetrician William Shippen, Jr., Morgan's bitter enemy; the physicians Thomas Bond and Thomas Cadwalader, who left an original treatise on the West India "dry gripes"; the anatomist Caspar Wistar; and the surgeon Philip Syng Physick.

The most famous American doctor of the time was Benjamin Rush (1745–1813), who after six years of apprenticeship with Dr. John Redman studied and graduated in Edinburgh. Rush, like Benjamin Franklin, was a typical representative of the Enlightenment. A signer of the Declaration of Independence, he espoused numerous "causes," including the emancipation of slaves, antialcoholism, the abolition of the death penalty, and money reform. His early interests in psychiatry and anthropology are typical of his breadth. Rush was a man of tremendous energy and a good clinical observer, although the title of "American Sydenham," bestowed upon him by devoted friends, is somewhat exaggerated. In the clinical field he was far more an eighteenth-century systematist than a follower of Sydenham. He produced a variation of John Brown's system, in which, as a consistent monotheist, he reduced the number of diseases from two to one. He also recommended a heroic application of bloodletting and purging which was no less murderous for being honest—he treated himself in this fashion. After the famous yellow fever epidemic in Philadelphia in 1793 Rush became the leader of the American anticontagionists.

Another fine medical center existed at Harvard University, attracting such men as Benjamin Waterhouse (1754–1846), who had studied in Edinburgh and Leyden. Waterhouse introduced vaccination in 1800, supported by the moral authority of Thomas Jefferson against considerable resistance. The third outstanding medical center of the period was New York, which could boast of men like Samuel Bard (1742–1821) and David Hosack (1769–1835), both Edinburgh students. Bard was physician to George Washington, and his treatise on diphtheria (1777) is regarded as a classic.

In the first decades of the nineteenth century American medical students started turning to Paris, the brilliant new metropolis of the medical world. Their favorite teacher was

Pierre Louis, the protagonist of clinical statistics. Although this French-trained group produced some outstanding men, it never exerted the large-scale influence of the earlier British- or later the German-trained group. This probably was due to the French group's orientation toward diagnosis and therapeutic skepticism, which were not congenial to the general utilitarian attitude in the United States. Louis trained such outstanding Philadelphia clinicians as Alfred Stillé (1813–1900), William Pepper (1810–1864), and William W. Gerhard (1809–1872). Gerhard made a great contribution to medical research when he definitely differentiated between typhoid fever and typhus in 1837. Other outstanding Philadelphia men of the period were the anatomist W. E. Horner (1793–1853), the great naturalist Joseph Leidy (1823–1891), and John K. Mitchell (1793–1858), the father of the neurologist Silas W. Mitchell. Mitchell propounded a fungus theory of malaria in 1849 which gained world-wide attention.

Of Louis' pupils in New England the best known are Oliver Wendell Holmes, whose work on puerperal fever has already been mentioned; Elisha Bartlett (1804–1855), the author of an excellent treatise on the fevers of the United States; Henry Ingersoll Bowditch (1808–1892), the great pioneer of public health; and Louis' favorite pupil James Jackson, Jr. (1810–1834), who died tragically young. Outstanding New England surgeons of the period were Paris-trained John Collins Warren (1778–1856), who performed the operation in which Morton publicly demonstrated his ether anesthesia, and Henry J. Bigelow (1818–1890), who reported it. The Paris school was ably represented in New York by Alonzo Clark (1807–1887).

The United States impressed the medical world during the first half of the nineteenth century by three major accomplishments. Its outstanding gynecological surgery has already been mentioned, with special reference to the first ovariotomies performed by Ephraim McDowell, himself an Edinburgh graduate. The invention of anesthesia has also been described earlier. The third important contribution was the research in stomach physiology carried out by William Beaumont (1785–1853) between 1822 and 1833.

American accomplishments in surgery and dentistry were a rather logical consequence of the particular conditions of the young country, besides being a reward for avoiding the separation of surgery and medicine. American surgeons like Sims, Mott, Bigelow, and Gross (who was also an outstanding pathologist) enjoyed an international reputation for their skill and daring. The physiological work of William Beaumont is one of the most admirable accomplishments in medical history. This simple tutor-trained military surgeon, who worked in the wilderness of the frontier, had the imagination to use the gastric fistula of one of his patients, Alexis St. Martin, for research in gastric physiology. Yet his achievement remained an isolated phenomenon for a long time. The time was not yet ripe for work in medical science in the United States. The early medical contributions of the growing frontier region of the Middle West were usually of a more practical nature. Typical are the outstanding clinical work of Austin Flint, Sr. (1812–1886) of Buffalo, the surgical and educational work of Daniel Brainerd (1812–1866) of Chicago, and the contributions to education and medical geography made by Daniel Drake (1785–1852). Drake's monumental treatise on *Diseases of the Interior Valley of North America* (1850–1854), based on thirty years of personal observations, is one of the classics of medical geography.

These outstanding accomplishments of American medicine in the first half of the nineteenth century unfortunately cannot obscure the fact that the situation as a whole grew increasingly unsatisfactory. The Civil War contributed to the decline, with the dissolution of the fine medical centers that had developed in the South, particularly in Virginia, Kentucky, Tennessee, and Louisiana. The rapid westward expansion of the country and the resulting absence of legal regulations lowered educational standards and gave free rein to ruthless commercialism. The old preceptorial training was now largely abandoned in favor of short courses in the proprietary schools that sprang up like mushrooms everywhere. The quality of these schools can easily be guessed from their numbers. There were no less than four hundred medical schools in the United States in the nineteenth century. Illinois had thirty-nine such schools, Missouri forty-two. In 1910 there were still one hundred and forty-eight medical schools left in the country, and it was not until 1930 that the number had been reduced to seventy-six well-qualified institutions. Sometimes diplomas were issued by "diploma mills" which did not pretend to give even the lowest grade of instruction.

Thus it was not the quantity of doctors which constituted a problem, but their quality. The public answered this development with a revolt, turning its confidence more and more toward such sectarian healers as the homeopaths and the eclectics. The better elements of the medical profession realized that some radical house cleaning was called for and founded the American Medical Association for this purpose in 1847. Medical education was also seriously hampered in the nineteenth century by the antidissection feeling of the people. This prejudice seems now largely overcome, though antivivisection fanatics still try to hamper medical research. Diffidence toward orthodox medicine was still strong enough in the second half of the nineteenth century to make possible the rise of sects such as Christian Science, osteopathy, and chiropractics.

The recovery of medicine in the last decades of the nineteenth century coincided with the rise to leadership of men trained in Germany or subjected to German influence, and with the concomitant introduction of laboratory medicine and training in the basic sciences. The recovery was spearheaded by the work of the Hopkins group and its "big four": William Osler (1847–1919), William S. Halsted (1852–1922), William H. Welch (1850–1934), and Howard Kelly (1858–1943). The Johns Hopkins Medical School, opening in Baltimore in 1893 as a full-fledged university department, exerted a tremendous influence upon American medical education. One of its leading figures, William "Popsy" Welch, had studied under Cohnheim and Ludwig, and at Hopkins he encouraged the emphasis on research methods and research facilities so typical of the German universities. Welch also was instrumental in formulating policy for the Rockefeller Foundation, founded in 1901, which was to play such a great role in the development and sponsoring of research in the United States.

Although Johns Hopkins played a dominant role in the reform of medical teaching in the United States, it is but fair to remember that several older schools had previously made serious efforts in this direction. Harvard had introduced a graded three-year course in 1871, Pennsylvania and Syracuse in 1877, and Michigan in 1880. Harvard made it possible in 1871 for Henry Pickering Bowditch (1840–1911), another pupil of Ludwig and a physiologist of international stature, to open a physiological laboratory. The great and immediate successes of the new medical sciences appealed to American utilitarianism and did much to reconcile the public with the medical profession. This was especially true for the discoveries of bacteriology, to which the United States contributed the outstanding work of Theobald Smith, Walter Reed, and Simon Flexner. Their accomplishments were followed by those of Ricketts, Rous, Ashburn, Zinsser, Theiler, and others. American contributions in the field of biochemistry are dealt with in Chapter 20. We might merely mention here O. Folin and D. van Slyke. American work in the field of genetics (Th. H. Morgan, C. E. McClung, H. J. Muller) was great. It occurred mostly after 1900, just as did the American contribution to public health.

The new research and the new medicine could come into their own in the United States only when the problem of regulating medical education, solved centuries earlier in Europe, could finally be settled. This was accomplished at the beginning of the twentieth century, primarily through the efforts of the American Medical Association and the

Rockefeller Foundation. The famous reports of Abraham Flexner played an important part in the reforms. Whether the recent attempts in the United States to solve certain problems of medical care through the creation of "barefoot-doctors" (physicians' aides, etc.) will be salutary, remains to be seen.

The story of American medicine during this period would not be complete without a mention of one more great accomplishment—the foundation of the Surgeon General's Library, which has become the greatest medical library in the world. In connection with this library two invaluable medical bibliographical tools have been developed: the Index Catalog of the Surgeon General's Library (now the National Library of Medicine), and the Quarterly Indexes. The remarkable growth of the Surgeon General's Library was largely due to the work of John Shaw Billings (1838–1913). Billings also played an important role in the founding of the Johns Hopkins Medical School, initiated many sanitary reforms, and revitalized the New York Public Library. A rather austere character who lacked the personal charm of the beloved "Popsy" Welch, he deserves a large share of the credit for the stimulation of American medical scholarship at the end of the nineteenth century and the beginning of the twentieth.

A natural result of stricter educational standards was the development of stricter licensing procedures, since medical schools were bound to be concerned with the competition their products faced from tutor-trained doctors and quacks. Effective state licensing bodies were generally instituted in the last decades of the nineteenth century. These reforms gave American medicine the strength it needed to play a leading role in world medicine. After the First World War American students no longer needed to go to Europe for postgraduate studies. Instead, Europeans tended more and more to come to the United States.

Chapter 20

EPILOGUE: TRENDS IN
TWENTIETH-CENTURY MEDICINE

Any survey of the achievements and trends of medicine during the present century cannot be historical in the same sense as were the earlier chapters of this book. The distance from events is too short, the personal involvements are too great, and the mass of data is too overpowering to allow a balanced judgment as to what is permanent and what is only of passing value in the accomplishments of the last fifty years. A similar chapter written sixty years ago, when the present author entered the field of medicine, would undoubtedly have emphasized events that are now long forgotten, while overlooking advances that have since proved to be of great importance and vitality. This chapter will, therefore, be weighed down with as few names and details as possible.

In spite of the unprecedented achievements of this century, some of the most prominent and "modern" traits of present-day medicine actually were already well in evidence in the nineteenth century. The development of endocrinology in the 1880's has already been described. Even a few endocrine extracts had been prepared in the nineteenth century, notably suprarenin by Oliver and Schaefer in 1894, and thyroiodin by Baumann in 1895. The greatest practical achievement to date in modern endocrinology was the isolation of insulin by F. G. Banting of Toronto and his co-workers in 1921, following the work of Paulesco, a discovery which resulted in a complete change in the prognosis for "incurable" diabetes. Meanwhile, insulin has been partly replaced by peroral drugs. Cortisone and ACTH have found a respected position in therapeutics, though they have not fulfilled all expectations originally uttered for them. E. C. Kendall of the Mayo Foundation isolated cortisone in 1939; he had isolated thyroxine in 1914. Endocrinology unexpectedly entered the field of cancer therapy with the work of Hughes (1941).

Of the more than twenty characteristic traits of modern preventive medicine given by Garrison (see his *History of Medicine* [4th edition], p. 670), there is hardly one that had not already been developed in principle by the nineteenth century. Differences between the preventive medicine of the nineteenth century and the twentieth century are more quantitative than qualitative. The present century saw the introduction of large-scale vaccination against diphtheria, tuberculosis, and tetanus, and successful campaigns were undertaken against yellow fever, malaria, smallpox, and hookworm all over the world. With the insecticide DDT, remarkable results in typhus prevention were obtained in the Second World War. The polio vaccines of Salk (1955) and Sabin (1956) yielded dramatic results. The complete inability of medicine to cope with the influenza epidemic of 1918, which with its twenty million victims destroyed more human lives than all the battles of the First World War, served both as a valuable stimulus and as a sobering influence. New discoveries in the thirties entirely changed the medical world's concepts of yellow fever and typhus. In spite of the continuous progress in microbiology, emphasis in preventive medicine grew less and less exclusively bacteriological. The trend toward social pathology, starting again with Grotjahn about 1900, has produced a new "social medicine" which has profoundly influenced thought in the field of preventive medicine.

X-rays have entirely transformed diagnostic techniques, and have become an important therapeutic agent. Yet x-rays were discovered by Wilhelm Konrad Roentgen (1845–1922) in 1895 and were immediately used for diagnostic purposes.

They were even applied to the gastro-intestinal tract before 1900 by Walter B. Cannon of Harvard. The use of x-ray and radium treatments had already been begun in the nineteenth century. Radium, which until recently has been the only other important element in radiation therapy, was discovered by the Curies in 1898. Recent progress in atomic research has brought other radioactive substances, the radioactive isotopes, into use in diagnostics and therapeutics. The whole field of diagnostics has made tremendous progress with an expanding technology from the electrocardiograph to ultrasound, tomography, and other applications of the computer. Among the diagnostic instruments actually invented in the twentieth century, the most important were the electrocardiograph, invented by Willem Einthoven of Leyden in 1903, and the electroencephalograph, developed by Hans Berger of Jena in 1929. Blood pressure apparati (Basch, 1881; Riva Rocci, 1897) existed in the nineteenth century. The rapidly increasing construction of medical machines (ultrasound, the pacemaker, tomography, dialysis, etc.) has produced a new branch of engineering: biomedical engineering.

Biochemistry at present affords one of the most common approaches to medical problems. Yet the trend toward biochemistry is by no means a child of the present century. Emil Fischer (1852–1919), with his synthesis of veronal (phenobarbital) and his work on sugars, nucleoproteids, amino acids, and polypeptides, might be regarded as representative of the more recent developments in biochemistry. Yet his work and his influence date from the 1870's. Most of the investigations by Fischer and his contemporaries centered round the problem of nutrition, and it was in the field of nutrition that one of the most significant contributions of the twentieth century was made. This was the discovery of vitamins.

The fact that synthetic diets lacked some essential factors was observed by Lunin in 1881. In 1882 Takaki's study of

Japanese naval personnel showed that a change in diet could prevent beriberi, the most prevalent avitaminosis of the Far East. As early as 1747 Lind had pointed out the importance of diet for the control of scurvy in the British navy. Through feeding experiments on chickens, using polished and unpolished rice, the Dutchman Christiaan Eijkman showed in 1897 that beriberi was due to the absence of minute amounts of unknown substances in the food. In 1906 Frederick G. Hopkins developed the concept of accessory foodstuffs, and Casimir Funk named them "vitamines" in 1912.

The United States achieved leadership in the field of vitamin research through the work of E. V. McCollum and Harry Steenbock at the University of Wisconsin and Thomas B. Osborn and L. B. Mendel at Yale. The Wisconsin and Yale groups discovered vitamin A in 1913 and vitamin B in 1916. In 1914 Goldberger's work identified pellagra as a B-deficiency disease. The German Huldschinsky demonstrated the antirachitic effect of ultraviolet light in 1919. McCollum and Steenbock discovered antirachitic vitamin D in 1922, and in 1924 the independent results of Hess and Steenbock showed that the antirachitic effect of ultraviolet light was due to the fact that it activated a provitamin into vitamin D. The German Windaus was able to identify this provitamin as ergosterol in 1927. Large-scale elimination of rickets has followed these discoveries, with a corresponding reduction of fatal accidents in childbirth. Meanwhile vitamin B has been broken down into different elements of a complex, vitamins C, K, and E have been added to the list, and the field of vitamin research has grown so tremendously that it is not feasible to give further details in a chapter primarily concerned with trends rather than individual achievements.

Vitamin research attracted few supporters in its infancy because of the dominance of bacteriology and the ensuing fixed idea that all diseases were the consequence of some kind of microbe action. It also ran counter to the crude quantitative ideas of nutrition prevailing at the time. But latterly vitamin research has branched out tremendously. It has enriched all fields of medicine, especially pediatrics. It has unfortunately also given rise to an extremely costly and medically unjustifiable attack on the pocketbooks of the gullible hypochondriacs who seem as common now as in former, less enlightened times. These disadvantages are minor compared to the benefits brought about by nutritional research (enzymes, trace elements, etc.) and nutritional improvement through greater diet consciousness. Somewhat related to the field of nutrition was the discovery made in 1926 by George Richards Minot that consumption of raw liver would effectively control pernicious anemia. If to these therapeutic accomplishments (sera, hormones, and vitamins, and, later, anticoagulants, found by K. P. Link and other United States biochemists), we add radiotherapy, chemotherapy, and surgery as described below, we are entitled to state that therapeutics achieved progress in the twentieth century comparable to that of pathology and prevention in the nineteenth century.

One of the most significant medical achievements of the present century is undoubtedly chemotherapy. The drugs of the past, synthetic or otherwise, had been largely symptomatic. The few specifics, such as quinine, had been found empirically, and their mode of action was unknown. But now drugs with a known action could be specifically compounded to fight diseases of known cause. The old ideal of drug treatment approached its fulfillment.

The new field grew primarily out of the labors of one great man, Paul Ehrlich (1854–1915). As a student, Ehrlich was intensely interested in staining methods, especially in vital stains. With his new staining methods he was able in the seventies and eighties to establish the present classification of leukocytes, thereby opening up the field of modern hematology. Clinically this field owes much to the work of Georges Hayem (1841–1933). His preoccupation with vital stains suggested to Ehrlich the famous side-chain theory. This theory, which holds that there is a special chemical affinity between certain drugs and certain cells, caused

Ehrlich to look for a chemical compound which would specifically bind and destroy the *Spirochaeta pallida* of syphilis while remaining sufficiently innocuous to the unhappy carrier of the spirochete. Work on the *Spirochaeta pallida* grew out of earlier, partly accidental observations that certain other spirochetes were particularly sensitive to dyes and their derivatives. After trying hundreds of chemical combinations, Ehrlich finally obtained an effective drug in 1910, with the help of his Japanese assistant Hata. This drug, first called "606" because it was the 606th combination tried, was later named salvarsan (arsphenamine). A less toxic combination, neosalvarsan (neoarsphenamine; drug no. 914), became the sovereign remedy for syphilis up to the discovery of penicillin. Out of Ehrlich's side-chain theory and Bordet's complement fixation test (1901) grew the serological test for syphilis found by Wassermann in 1906.

Ehrlich was a prolific worker. Besides his biochemical research, he carried out important studies on immunity, cancer, and urine reactions. And the influence of his fertile mind was even more significant than his immediate practical achievements. Nonetheless, during the twenty years following Ehrlich's death—called by Galdston the "doldrum years" of chemotherapy—the field lay barren and was almost abandoned as hopeless. The only important drugs found during this period were the antiplasmodials atabrine and plasmochin, both directed against malaria. It seemed impossible to find effective antibacterial drugs. The picture changed suddenly with the introduction of the sulfa drugs, also derivatives of dyes, by Gerhart Domagk in 1935. A new era of hope, discovery, and success began for chemotherapy. The sulfa drugs were to a certain extent superseded in the early forties by penicillin and related drugs, now usually referred to as antibiotics. Penicillin, as is well known, is a mold product with a bactericidal effect. The bactericidal effect of molds has been known since the time of Pasteur, and attempts to derive drugs from molds were frequent toward the end of the nineteenth century. Typical were the experiments with pyocyanase in 1899 and Gosio's experiments with *Penicillium* in 1896. These experiments were abandoned because of lack of funds, and after these early trials the field was given up as apparently barren.

The new work with penicillin goes back to a chance observation by Sir Alexander Fleming in 1929. The practical development of the drug was accomplished by Florey and Chain in England in 1939. Since that time other antibiotics, such as streptomycin, aureomycin, and chloromycetin, have been prepared from molds. The sulfa drugs and penicillin have made it possible to deal successfully with infections caused by streptococci, (septicemia and puerperal fever), staphylococci, meningococci, gonococci, and pneumococci. The newer antibiotics have brought the plague and Koch's bacillus, and even rickettsias, within reach of the therapist. These drugs still seem to be ineffective in most of the virus diseases. There is also an alarming new "hospitalism," which is produced by bacteria that have become resistant to antibiotics. The progress, unimaginable to anyone who has not witnessed the miseries of the preantibiotic era, is nevertheless immense. With the increasing role of virus—especially slow virus—diseases, the need for antivirus drugs has become increasingly urgent.

It is quite possible that the dominant position of biochemistry will be challenged by biophysics, and that the more recent fundamental changes in physics will eventually bring about completely new approaches and methods in medicine. Yet the first applications of the new physics, in the form of tracer elements and isotopes, are too recent to allow any appraisal of their results here.

Allergic diseases, the so-called "idiosyncracies," have been observed by clinicians ever since the seventeenth century, with special attention being given to asthma. But it was left to the twentieth century to recognize the interrelatedness of these diseases and their underlying mechanisms. To this time too belongs the elaboration of efficient therapeutic methods like desensitization and antihistamines

(D. Bovet, 1937; Halpern, 1942). These insights grew out of the studies of Charles Richet (1903) and Theobald Smith (1902) on the phenomenon of anaphylaxis. The term "allergy" was coined by Clemens von Pirquet in 1903.

The term "geriatrics" was first used by the American, Nascher, in 1916, and at first sight this specialty appears to be a twentieth-century development. Yet preoccupation with the diseases of old age is nothing new in medicine. It can be seen in the works of Hippocrates as well as in the medieval search for the "elixir" of life. It appears in a more rational form in the Renaissance treatise of Luigi Cornaro (1467–1566), and an extensive literature on the subject existed in the eighteenth century. The present-day approach was outlined as early as 1867 in Charcot's classic book, which discussed the various diseases of old age according to organs, applying pathological-anatomical data at the level of knowledge of the time. The modern approach, like Charcot's, still lacks any fundamental notion of the distinction between normal and pathological changes in old age.

Increased knowledge of cancer and other diseases has naturally aided the cause of geriatrics. Between 1940 and 1970, cancer mortality has been considerably reduced by a combination of improved surgery, radiation, and chemotherapy. Particularly valuable were the studies of hypertension by such men as Huchard, Allbutt, and von Basch in the 1880's. Bacteriology, endocrinology, and all the other new medical specialties of the last two generations have also made important contributions. Nevertheless, the primary stimulus to the current emphasis on diseases of old age has come, not from any new medical discoveries, but from a social situation. Because of the decreasing birth rate and the increasing life expectancy, the proportion of middle-aged and old people in all the Western nations is growing rapidly. In the United States people over forty-five now form one-third of the population, while at the turn of the century they formed only one-fifth and a hundred years ago only one-eighth of the population.

Mental disease has also become an increasingly acute problem of modern society, and the physical treatment of it has made important progress during the twentieth century. The malaria treatment, introduced by Wagner-Jauregg of Vienna in 1917 after forty years of research, has proved effective in reducing the damage done by general paresis. As in the case of arsphenamine, it has now largely been superseded by penicillin treatment.

During the 1930's, shock treatment and so-called psychosurgery were introduced in schizophrenia and depressions, i.e., psychoses of unknown origin. Reports of successes were undoubtedly often exaggerated. Fortunately the "psychopharmacy" (Serpasil, chlorpromazine, and so on) appearing during the 1950's has made it possible to forego these rather brutal methods. The tranquilizers have, in quieting down the excited patient, completely changed the physiognomy of mental institutions. Psychotherapeutic trends in the twentieth century have been reported in a previous chapter.

Another medical trend has gained momentum during the last decade under the name of "psychosomatic medicine." Psychosomatic medicine deals primarily with the psychological elements in bodily diseases or complaints. With all due sympathy for this very worth-while undertaking, the medical historian is obliged to state that the discoveries of psychosomatic medicine are often only rediscoveries, not always improved by the use of a somewhat fanciful nomenclature. The fact that bodily diseases or symptoms are profoundly influenced by mental processes, often partially caused by them, was well known to all great clinicians from Erasistros and Galen to Charcot and Struempell. Psychogenesis, or "passion-produced disease," as Galen called it, was thus discussed abundantly until the nineteenth century. There were erroneous psychogenic explanations, like that of plague (Paracelsus, Stahl, or Van Swieten), typhus, rabies, tuberculosis, and cancer (in the nineteenth century). The last such occurrence was the labeling of New Guinea's kuru as psychogenic in 1958, five years before Gajdusek isolated the slow virus that caused it. It seems unlikely that the new trend is primarily due to any recent increase in the incidence of this type of complaint. What appears to have happened is that in the latter part of the nineteenth century and the first half of the twentieth century the old insights were lost in the shuffle of fascinating objective discoveries with the attendant over-mechanization and overspecialization. Doctors became so laboratory-minded, so scientific, and so impersonal, that they forgot, or felt entitled to ignore, the patient as a person. It is a queer reflection on the present age that one of the basic medical functions of all times now had to be reintroduced—as a new specialty. This new trend profited from our affluent society's overwhelming preoccupation with psychology, aptly labeled in medical terms as "iatropsychology" by Jerome Schneck (1961).

Meanwhile, specialization has spread continuously. The American medical directory now lists sixty-six specialties, the last of which is aerospace medicine. Nineteenth-century "internal medicine" has split into such fields of specialization as cardiovascular diseases, pulmonary diseases, endocrinology, hematology, gastrointestinal diseases, nephrology, etc. Pediatrics has split along similar lines, as has surgery.

Other social problems of twentieth-century medicine, like increases in the cost of medical care, hospitals, auxiliaries, insurance systems, and group practice, have been dealt with in chapters 17 and 18.

Surgery has continued its brilliant advance in the twentieth century. The sharp lines of separation between surgery and internal medicine have fortunately tended more and more to disappear as a result of closer collaboration and the increasing reliance of both on a common grounding in the basic sciences. Surgeons have become interested in medical problems, and physicians, particularly neurologists, have sometimes developed into surgeons. The care of some conditions, such as hyperthyroidism and peptic ulcers, has alternated between the provinces of surgery and medicine, as each branch in turn has been able to offer more effective methods of control.

Surgery has made its main advances during the current century in its work on the chest, the brain, and the sympathetic system. Chest surgery can be said to have started with the introduction of pneumothorax work by Forlanini in 1882, and its beginnings are closely connected with the name of Ferdinand Sauerbruch (1875–1951). In the 1940's, heart surgery was added through the work of R. E. Gross, Crafoord, and A. Blalock. Horsley, Broca, and others performed brain operations in the nineteenth century, but brain surgery achieved the stature of a discipline through the work of Harvey Cushing (1869–1939) and Walter Dandy (1886–1946). Surgery of the sympathetic system owes much to René Leriche and M. Jabouley. Transfusion experiments have been made ever since Richard Lower's attempt in 1665, but transfusion could only become safe as a valuable routine procedure after the discovery of the blood groups by Karl Landsteiner of Vienna in 1901. Progress in anesthesia is, next to that in transfusion, at the root of recent gains in surgery. Modern intensive care units are often developed by anesthetists. A tremendously important new field of surgery —organ transplantation—opened up with large-scale kidney transplants (beginning with Murray, Hamburger, Storze, and others) in the 1960's. Experimental work in this field goes back to the beginning of our century. Because of organ transplantation, death has been redefined as electroencephalographic demonstration of brain death. Along with the spectacular feats of brain and thorax surgery, the solid accomplishments of orthopedics, such as prosthetic joint replacement, should not be overlooked.

In spite of their alleged indifference toward general principles, medical scientists have never entirely ceased to search for them. After the middle of the nineteenth century solidistic pathology seemed to have ruled out humoral pathology entirely; but the humoralistic view was granted an unexpected rejuvenation by the discoveries of endocrinology. After their discovery of secretin in 1902, two British endocrinologists, Bayliss and Starling, propounded the theory that "hormones" controlled the functions of the body. The solidistic point of view gained ground again with the work of Eppinger and Hess (1910) on vagotony and sympathicotony, as a result of which they held the function of the endocrine glands to be under the direction of the vegetative nervous system. Eppinger and Hess were able to present this point of view on the basis of an extensive study of the vegetative system made by the English physiologists Gaskell, Langley, and Sherrington. The greater part of this study was carried out toward the end of the nineteenth century. During the same period Ivan Petrovich Pavlov (1849–1936) started publishing his experiments on conditional reflexes, which have had a tremendous influence on medical and psychological thought, especially in Russia and Russian-controlled countries. Numerous attacks from the camp of humoralists were largely invalidated by the studies of Metchnikoff and Aschoff on the role of the reticulo-endothelial system. The work of H. Selye gave a new impetus to humoralism.

In the recent past the field of constitution has not always attracted the well-deserved attention given to it by earlier practitioners. Progress in genetics in the twentieth century, combined with new experience in the area of internal secretions, has once again stimulated interest in the influence of hereditary make-up on the evolution of disease in the individual. Constitution studies developed as a reaction against bacteriology, as the realization grew that the "soil," as well as the "seed," was important in infectious disease. These studies were also a reaction against the extreme localism of the nineteenth century. They appealed to men like the clinician Friedrich Kraus (1858–1936), who saw in them a return to approaching the patient as a whole personality rather than a mere conglomeration of organs. It is quite possible that constitution studies may in the future acquire greater importance than they have had in the past.

It is possible that a synthesis of genetics and biochemistry as it has developed in so-called "molecular pathology" will also explain a great number of pathological processes. This trend started with the work of Archibald Garrod (1857–1936) on the "inborn errors of metabolism." Since then, it has been possible to explain a number of diseases through faulty formation and transformation of molecules; e.g., different forms of inability to decompose phenylalanine can result in idiocy, or aecaptonuria, or albinism. These genetic studies are of better quality than the stopgap diagnoses for cases of leprosy, scabies, rickets, puerperal fever, pellagra, general paresis, and others, made a hundred years ago and regarded then as hereditary. Genetics became a scientific discipline only with the work of Gregory Mendel (1822–1884), first published in 1865 and rediscovered in 1900.

As a whole, medical progress during the last fifty years has been stupendous. Of course, the elimination of so many infections, with the consequent prolongation of the average life by decades, has led to an unprecedented prevalence of cancer and degenerative cardiovascular diseases against which so far medicine's ability to fight successfully is rather limited. Then there is the appalling fact that so many lives are saved by medicine only to be lost through accidents. Accidents are a terrible load on our surgeons and hospitals, and have brought into being the field of traumatology, which is very important in the medicine of catastrophes. One could argue that, at least in Western countries, where the financial order is represented by increased longevity and the omnipresence of the automobile, we have progressed from diseases of poverty to diseases of affluence. The present accident rate is such that more years could be added to the average life expectancy by the elimination of accidents than by extirpation of cancer and tuberculosis combined! And those who boast of medical progress might well remember that even now no answer can be given to a question asked by Jakob Henle more than a hundred years ago: "Has anybody something better to offer than words when it comes to the proximate causes of rheumatism, hysteria, and cancer?" But on the whole an examination of the medical history of the last seventy-five years, especially as seen against the background of earlier centuries, cannot but lead to a great satisfaction and even greater hopes.

Paradoxically, doctors have not become more popular through their improved means of helping. The perennial ambivalence of the patient, always in search of a scapegoat, has, with the help of quacks, politicians, and sensation-mongering mass media, increased. The patient and his family, depressed through weakness and a sense of helplessness, can easily misinterpret as callous the conventional doctor's dispassionate search for a diagnosis. The quack, who can neither diagnose nor recommend objective therapy, is often more reassuring with his irresponsible chatter.

Sometimes the doctor himself becomes a quack. The beautiful dream of the enlightenment—that with the growth of science, superstition will disappear—has not come true. Superstition has become more sophisticated, but our society is submerged by it and our contemporaries are steeped in it. It is with us as much as it was in ancient Rome or in seventeenth-century Europe. Every swindle with the prefix "bio," every "millennial wisdom" from the East, every psychological absurdity or PSI has legions of enthusiasts. Why shouldn't doctors, who are no less suggestible than their patients, join them on the path of unscientific "science?"

The advances of the last two centuries have made the doctor a far happier man than was his predecessor. His powers to prevent and control disease have grown out of all recognition. If scientific progress can be kept at present levels—which is no foregone conclusion but needs untiring and intelligent efforts; if the social gap can be bridged between medical knowledge and its availability to the majority of the community; if civilization is able to survive the catastrophies which threaten it; then most of the history of medicine so far may be hardly more than "prehistory" to future historians and doctors. Yet their debt to their predecessors will be as immeasurable as is ours to the anonymous caveman who once in the dim past discovered the use of fire.

NOBEL LAUREATES IN MEDICINE AND PHYSIOLOGY, 1901- 1981

The trends of twentieth-century medicine are relatively well illustrated by the names of those who received the Nobel Prize in Medicine and Physiology from its foundation to the present. We give therefore in the following a list of the Nobel Laureates in medicine and physiology between 1901 and 1981.

1901 EMIL VON BEHRING, serum therapy against diphtheria.

1902 RONALD ROSS, discovery of life cycle of causative agent of malaria.

1903 NIELS RYBERG FINSEN, phototherapy for lupus vulgaris.

1904 IVAN PETROVICH PAVLOV, studies of digestion physiology.

1905 ROBERT KOCH, work on tuberculosis; development of scientific bacteriology.

1906 CAMILLO GOLGI, SANTIAGO RAMÓN Y CAJAL, work on structure of nervous system.

1907 CHARLES LOUIS ALPHONSE LAVERAN, studies of protozoa.

1908 PAUL EHRLICH, ELIE METCHNIKOFF, work on immunity.

1909 EMIL THEODOR KOCHER, work on physiology, pathology, and surgery of thyroid gland.

1910 ALBRECHT KOSSEL, studies in cellular chemistry.

1911 ALLVAR GULLSTRAND, work on dioptrics of the eye.

1912 ALEXIS CARREL, development of methods for vascular ligature and grafting of blood vessels and organs.

1913 CHARLES RICHET, development of anaphylaxis.

1914 ROBERT BÁRÁNY, studies of vestibular system.

1915–1918 (No awards.)

1919 JULES BORDET, work on immunity.

1920 SCHACK AUGUST STEENBERG KROGH, discovery of mechanism regulating capillaries.

1921 (No award.)

1922 ARCHIBALD VIVIAN HILL, OTTO FRITZ MEYERHOF, work on biochemistry of muscle.

1923 FREDERICK GRANT BANTING, JOHN JAMES RICKARD MACLEOD, discovery of insulin.

1924 WILLEM EINTHOVEN, invention and development of electro-cardiograph.

1925 (No award.)

1926 JOHANNES ANDREAS GRIB FIBIGER, discovery of spiroptera carcinoma.

1927 JULIUS WAGNER-JAUREGG, malaria inoculation in treatment of paresis.

1928 CHARLES NICOLLE, work on typhus exanthematicus.

1929 CHRISTIAAN EIJKMAN, FREDERICK GOWLAND HOPKINS, discoveries of vitamins.

1930 KARL LANDSTEINER, discovery of human blood groups.

1931 OTTO HEINRICH WARBURG, work on respiratory enzyme.

1932 CHARLES SCOTT SHERRINGTON, EDGAR DOUGLAS ADRIAN, work on function of the neuron.

1933 THOMAS HUNT MORGAN, work on hereditary function of chromosomes.

1934 GEORGE RICHARDS MINOT, WILLIAM PARRY MURPHY, GEORGE HOYT WHIPPLE, liver treatment of pernicious anemia.

1935 HANS SPEMANN, work in experimental embryology.

1936 HENRY HALLETT DALE, OTTO LOEWI, research on chemical transmission of nerve impulses.

1937 ALBERT VON SZENT-GYÖRGYI VON NAGYRAPOLT, work on biological oxidation, especially vitamin C and catalysis of fumaric acid.

1938 CORNEILLE HEYMANS, work on central regulation of respiration.

1939 GERHARD DOMAGK, discovery of antibacterial effect of prontociliate.

1940–1942 (No awards.)

1943 HENRIK DAM, EDWARD ADELBERT DOISY, discovery and analysis of vitamin K.

1944 JOSEPH ERLANGER, HERBERT SPENCER GASSER, work on changes in electric potential of nerve fibers.

1945 ALEXANDER FLEMING, ERNST BORIS CHAIN, HOWARD WALTER FLOREY, discovery of penicillin.

1946 HERMANN JOSEPH MULLER, study of mutation through irradiation.

1947 CARL FERDINAND CORI, GERTY THERESA CORI, work on glycogen metabolism.

BERNARDO ALBERTO HOUSSAY, study of hormone of anterior lobe of hypophysis.

1948   PAUL MUELLER, discovery of insect-killing properties of DDT.

1949   WALTER RUDOLF HESS, work on midbrain.

ANTONIO CAETANO DE ABREU FREIRE EGAS MONIZ, development of prefrontal leucotomy.

1950   PHILIP SHOWALTER HENCH, EDWARD CALVIN KENDALL, TADEUSZ REICHSTEIN, discoveries about hormones of adrenal cortex, *e.g.* cortisone.

1951   MAX THEILER, development of anti-yellow-fever vaccine.

1952   SELMAN ABRAHAM WAKSMAN, co-discovery of streptomycin.

1953   FRITZ ALBERT LIPMANN, discovery of coenzyme A.

HANS ADOLPH KREBS, discovery of citric-acid cycle.

1954   JOHN FRANKLIN ENDERS, THOMAS HUCKLE WELLER, FREDERICK CHAPMAN ROBBINS, work with cultivation of polio virus in human tissues.

1955   AXEL HUGO THEORELL, work on enzymes of oxidation.

1956   DICKINSON W. RICHARDS, JR., ANDRÉ F. COURNAND, WERNER FORSSMANN, development of new techniques in treating heart disease.

1957   DANIEL BOVET, development of drugs to relieve allergies and relax muscles during surgery.

1958   JOSHUA LEDERBERG, GEORGE WELLS BEADLE, EDWARD LAWRIE TATUM, work on chemistry of genes.

1959   SEVERO OCHOA, ARTHUR KORNBERG, discoveries on mechanism of synthesis of ribonucleic and deoxyribonucleic acids.

1960   FRANK MACFARLANE BURNET, PETER BRIAN MEDAWAR, studies of acquired immunological tolerance.

1961   GEORG VON BEKESY, discoveries concerning mechanism of hearing.

1962   FRANCIS COMPTON CRICK, JAMES DEWEY WATSON, MAURICE HUGH FREDERICK WILKINS, elucidation of three-dimensional molecular structure of DNA.

1963   ALAN LLOYD HODGKIN, ANDREW FIELDING HUXLEY, JOHN CAREW ECCLES, work on ion transfer in nervous stimulation.

1964   KONRAD E. BLOCH, FEODOR LYNEN, work on control of cholesterol.

1965   FRANÇOIS JACOB, ANDRÉ LWOFF, JACQUES MONOD, work on genetics of bacteria.

1966   CHARLES BRENTON HUGGINS, FRANCIS PEYTON ROUS, work on the genesis and chemical control of cancer.

1967   HALDAN KESSER HARTLINE, GEORGE WALD, RAGNAR GRANIT, discoveries concerning physiology and chemistry of sight.

1968   ROBERT W. HOLLEY, HAR GOBAND KORANA, MARSHALL W. NIRENBERG, interpretation of genetic codes in protein synthesis.

1969 MAX DELBRÜCK, ALFRED D. HERSHEY, SALVADOR E. LURIA, genetic structure of virus.

1970 JULIUS AXELROD, ULF VON EULER, BERNHARD KATZ, humoral transmission in nerves.

1971 EARL WILBUR SUTHERLAND, JR., mechanisms of hormone action.

1972 GERALD M. EDELMAN, RODNEY R. PORTER, chemical structures of antibodies.

1973 KARL VON FRISCH, KONRAD LORENZ, NIKOLAAS TINBERGEN, behavior in animals.

1974 ALBERT CLAUDE, CHRISTIAN DE DUVE, GEORGE E. PALADE, cell structure and function.

1975 DAVID BALTIMORE, RENATO DULBECCO, HOWARD TEMIN, interaction of tumor virus and genetic material.

1976 BARUCH S. BLUMBERG, DANIEL CARLETON GAJDUSEK, virus of hepatitis and Kuru.

1977 ROSALYN S. YALOW, radioimmune essay.
ROGER C. L. GUILLEMIN, ANDREW V. SCHALLY, hormone formation in the brain.

1978 WERNER ARBER, HAMILTON SMITH, DANIEL NATHANS, restrictive enzymes.

1979 ALLAN MCLEOD CORMAK, GODFREY NEWBOLD HOUNSFIELD, computerized tomography.

1980 JEAN DAUSSAT, BARUJ BENCERRAF, GEORGE SNELL, genetic control of immunity.

1981 ROGER W. SPERRY, specialized functions of cerebral hemispheres.
DAVID H. HUBEL, TORSTEN N. WEISEL, information processing in the visual system.

SUGGESTIONS FOR FURTHER READING

In this short book the author has deliberately limited himself to a bare outline of the history of medicine. Material which merits a book in itself has often been compressed into a paragraph. For the reader who has become intrigued with some particular period, technical development, problem, or person, a bibliographical guide is offered for each of the chapters.

The author would like to call particular attention to the translations and reprints listed for appropriate chapters. He believes these original classics—reflecting the essence of history—often make more interesting and provocative reading than even good books "about" the classics. For those who do not have access to these reprints and translations of original books, source books are available which present at least snippets of the original material. Two good source books are R. H. Major (ed.), *Classic Descriptions of Disease* (Springfield, Ill., 1945) and F. A. Willius and Thomas E. Keys (eds.), *Cardiac Classics* (St. Louis, 1941). The last has been reprinted by Dover Publications, Inc. (New York, 1961). Also highly recommended is C. N. B. Camac's *Classics of Medicine*, an anthology containing works of Lister, Harvey, Auenbrugger, Laennec, Jenner, Morton, Simpson, and Holmes, reprinted by Dover (New York, 1959) and L. Clendening, *Sourcebook in Medical History* (Dover Reprint, 60).

As reference works and for a more detailed study of a particular facet of medical history, the author recommends above all: F. H. Garrison, *Introduction to the History of Medicine* (4th ed.; Philadelphia, 1929); Max Neuburger, *History of Medicine*, English translation (London, 1910) (this work was unfortunately never finished and ends with the Middle Ages); Volumes I and II of H. E. Sigerist, *A History of Medicine* (New York, 1951); Emerson C. Kelly, *Encyclopedia of Medical Sources* (Baltimore, 1948); and Th. Puschmann, *A History of Medical Education* (1891; reprint 1966 by Hafner Publishing Co., The New York Academy of Medicine "History of Medicine Series," No. 28—abbreviated hereafter as Hafner). The only more recent good handbook is *Historia Universal de la Medicina*, edited by Pedro Lain Entralgo, 8 vols. (Barcelona, 1973). An English translation has been announced.

Biographical information concerning doctors of the United States is competently provided in the *Dictionary of American Medical Biography*, edited by H. A. Kelly and W. L. Burrage (New York, 1928). On an international scale such information can be found only in the two marvelous German publications: A. HIRSCH, E. GURLT, *et al., Biographisches Lexikon der hervorragenden Aerzte aller Laender und Zeiten* (5 vols., Berlin, 1929) and I. FISCHER, *Biographisches Lexikon der hervorragenden Aerzte der letzten fuenfzig Jahre* (Berlin, 1932).

For information on the history of diseases, consult A. HIRSCH, *Handbook of Geographical and Historical Pathology*, English translation, New Sydenham Society Publication (hereafter cited NSSP) No. 106 (3 vols., London, 1883); H. H. SCOTT, *A History of Tropical Medicine* (2 vols., Baltimore, 1939); and E. RODENWALT, *World Atlas of Epidemics* (Hamburg, 1952); and ERWIN H. ACKERKNECHT, *History and Geography of the Most Important Diseases* (New York, 1966).

Other "longitudinal sections" I recommend are O. WANGENSTEEN and S. WANGENSTEEN, *The Rise of Surgery* (Folkestone, 1978); G. MAJNO, *The Healing Hand* (Boston, 1975); ERWIN H. ACKERKNECHT, *Therapeutics from the Primitives to the 20th Century* (New York, 1973); KREMERS and URDANG, *History of Pharmacy*, revised by G. SONNEDECKER (Philadelphia, 1963); and W. WEINBERGER, *History of Dentistry* (St. Louis, 1948).

For those who have to obtain still more historical details on a given problem or person than those reference books can provide, the following procedure should prove of practical value:

1. Consult the catalog of your local library. That might lead you to a monograph or biography containing further bibliographical clues.

2. Consult the bibliography in Garrison's *Introduction*.

3. Look up *A Medical Bibliography* by F. H. GARRISON and L. T. MORTON (London, 1954). If you still need further information:

4. Look up the four series of the catalog of the Surgeon General's (now Armed Forces Medical) Library, our greatest reference tool in medicine and medical history.

There are three medical history periodicals in English: the *Bulletin of the History of Medicine, Medical History,* and the *Journal of the History of Medicine,* the occasional reading of which could be a relatively easy and pleasant way to become more familiar with the field. Also excellent reading is H. E. SIGERIST's history of medicine in biographical form: *The Great Doctors* (New York, 1933). A wealth of information is buried in the volumes of the now extinct *Annals of Medical History* and *Medical Life.* The former is very adequately indexed; the latter contains at least a list (in the last volume) of all articles published.

Specialized bibliographies the author would recommend here are A. L. BLOOMFIELD, *A Bibliography of Internal Medicine: Communicable Diseases* (Chicago, 1958), *Selected Diseases* (Chicago, 1960); and J. B. GILBERT, *Disease and Destiny, A Bibliography of Medical References to the Famous* (London, 1962).

CHAPTER 1

An excellent extensive survey of paleopathology is given in the first volume of H. E. SIGERIST, *History of Medicine* (New York, 1951). Sigerist also has an excellent, up-to-date bibliography, supplementing the extensive ones found in the classic treatises of R. L. MOODIE, *Paleopathology* (Chicago, 1923) and L. PALES, *Paléopathologie* (Paris, 1930). See also D. A. BROTHWELL and T. A. SANDISON, *Disease in Antiquity* (Springfield, 1963); and S. JARCHO, *Human Paleopathology* (New Haven, 1966).

CHAPTER 2

While there are no good modern monographs on primitive medicine, D. McKENZIE, *The Infancy of Medicine* (London, 1927) is relatively satisfactory. SIGERIST gives a competent survey in Volume I of his *History of Medicine*. See also a number of papers which this author has published in the *Bulletin of the History of Medicine*.

For a concrete picture of the medicine of individual primitive tribes the author recommends M. J. FIELD, *Religion and Medicine of the Ga People* (London, 1937); G. W. HARLEY, *Native African Medicine* (Cambridge, Mass., 1941); and the Cherokee study of J. MOONEY, *The Swimmer Manuscript*, revised and edited by FRANS OLBRECHTS (Smithsonian Institute, Bureau of American Ethnology Bull. No. 99; Washington, D.C., 1932). See also two sourcebooks in medical anthropology: D. LANDY, *Culture, Disease, and Healing* (New York, 1972); M. H. LOGAN and E. E. HUNT, *Health and the Human Condition* (North Scituate, 1978).

CHAPTER 3

There is no satisfactory monograph of any of the four medicines discussed in this chapter. SIGERIST gives excellent surveys of Egyptian and Mesopotamian medicine in the first volume of his *History of Medicine*.

There are good English editions of the *Edwin Smith Papyrus*, translated by J. H. BREASTED (2 vols., Chicago, 1930) and of the *Ebers Papyrus*, translated by B. EBBELL (Copenhagen, 1937). Numerous Mesopotamian texts have been published by R. CAMPBELL THOMPSON, especially in *Devils and Evil Spirits of Babylonia* (London, 1903) and in *Assyrian Medical Texts* (London, 1923).

For Mexico, see E. W. EMMART, *The Badianus Manuscript, An Aztec Herbal of 1552* (Baltimore, 1940).

CHAPTER 4

For a good survey of Hindu medicine, consult H. R. ZIMMER, *Hindu Medicine* (Baltimore, 1948) and also see the Hindu medical classic *Susruta Samhita*, translated by BHISHAGRATNA (3 vols., Calcutta, 1907–16), and *Charaka Samhita*, translated by CHANDRA KAOWARTE (Calcutta).

For Chinese medicine see E. H. Hume, *The Chinese Way of Medicine* (Baltimore, 1940) and Ilza Veith's translation of the first 34 chapters of Huang Ti nei ching su wen, *The Yellow Emperor's Classic of Internal Medicine* (Baltimore, 1949). A concise survey of both Chinese and Hindu medicine appears in the first volume of Neuburger's *History*. See also Wong and Wu, *History of Chinese Medicine* (Tientsin, 1932); and *The Barefoot Doctor's Manual* (Philadelphia, 1977).

Chapters 5, 6, and 7

Two good short surveys of Greek medicine are Henry Taylor Osborn, *Greek Biology and Medicine* (New York, n.d.) and Charles Singer, *Greek Biology and Medicine* (Oxford, 1922). For Greek religious medicine see W. A. Jayne, *The Healing Gods of Ancient Civilizations* (New Haven, 1925) and E. J. and L. Edelstein, *Asclepius* (2 vols., Baltimore, 1945). An excellent study of a specialized aspect is Sir Thomas Clifford Allbutt, *Greek Medicine in Rome* (London, 1921). A classic is O. Temkin, *Galenism* (Ithaca, 1973). Two source books are A. J. Brock, *Greek Medicine* (London, 1929) and M. R. Cohen and I. E. Drabkin, *A Sourcebook in Greek Science* (New York, 1948). The chapters in Neuburger, *History* remain the best written on this subject.

Translations

Anonymus Londonensis, The Medical Writings of. Trans. by W. H. S. Jones. Cambridge, 1947.

Aretaeus, The Extant Works of. Trans. by Francis Adams. (SSP No. 37.) London, 1856.

Asclepiades, Life and Writings. Trans. by R. M. Green. New Haven, 1955.

Caelius Aurelianus. *On Acute and on Chronic Diseases.* Trans. by I. E. Drabkin. Chicago, 1950.

Celsus. *De Medicina.* Trans. by W. G. Spencer. 3 vols. London, 1935–1938.

Dioscorides. *De materia medica.* Trans. by J. Goodyer. Oxford, 1934.

Frontinus, Sextus Junius. *On the Water Supply of the City of Rome.* Trans. by C. Herschel. Boston, 1899.

Galen. *Hygiene.* Trans. by R. M. Green. Springfield, 1951.

———. *On Anatomical Procedures.* Trans. by C. Singer. London, 1956.

———. *On Medical Experience.* Trans. by R. Walzer. London, 1947.

———. *On the Natural Faculties.* Trans. by A. J. Brock. London, 1916.

———. *Prognostics.* Trans. by M. Nutton. Berlin, 1979.

———. *On the Use of the Parts.* Trans. by M. T. May. Ithaca, 1968.

Hippocrates. Trans. by W. H. S. Jones. 4 vols. London, 1923–1931.

Soranus. *Gyneology.* Trans. by Owsei Temkin. Baltimore, 1956.

Chapter 8

For a general survey of this period consult David Riesman, *The Story of Medicine in the Middle Ages* (New York, 1935). Sir Thomas Clifford Allbutt has written a number of interesting essays on particular aspects of medieval medicine which are to be found in his *Science and Medieval Thought* (London, 1901) and *The Historical Relations of Medicine and Surgery* (London, 1905). An excellent survey of Arabian medicine is found in E. G. Browne, *Arabian Medicine* (Cambridge, 1921). Volume I of Lynn Thorndike's monumental, multi-volume *A History of Magic and Experimental Science* (New York, 1923) contains interesting and often entertaining material for this period. There have been many books written on the great plagues of this time, the most recent of which are Ph. Ziegler, *Black Death* (London, 1969); W. M. Bowsky, *Black Death* (New York, 1971).

Translations

Abulcasim. *On Surgery.* London, 1973.

Al Kindi. *Formulary.* Madison, 1966.

Avicenna. *The First Book of the Canon.* Trans. by O. C. Gruner. London, 1930.

Chauliac, Guy de. *On Wounds and Fractures.* Trans. by W. A. Brennan. Chicago, 1923.

Cockayne, Rev. O. (ed.). *Leechdoms, Wortcunning, and Starcraft of Early England.* 3 vols. London, 1864.

Dawson, W. R. *A Leechbook or Collection of Medical Recipes of the 15th Century* (Ms. No. 136 of the Medical Society of London). London, 1934.

Isidore of Sevilla: The Medical Writings. Trans. by W. D. Sharpe. Philadelphia, 1964.

John of Arderne. *De Arte Phisicale.* Trans. by Sir D'Arcy Power. New York, 1924.

Johannes de Mirfeld. *Breviarium Bartholomi et Florarium Bartholomi.* Trans. by Sir Percival Horton-Smith Hartley and H. R. Aldridge. Cambridge, 1936.

Ketham, J. *The fasciculus medicinae.* Trans. by Charles Singer. Milan, 1924.

Maimonides. *Treatise on Asthma.* Trans. by Suessmann Muntner. Philadelphia, 1963.

———. *Preservation of Youth.* Trans. by H. L. Gordon. New York, 1958.

Mondino. *Anothomia.* Trans. by Charles Singer. Florence, 1925.

Paulus of Aegineta, The Seven Books of. Trans. by Francis Adams. 3 vols. (SSP No. 4.) London, 1844.

RHAZES. *A Treatise on the Small Pox and Measles.* Trans. by A. GREENHILL. (SSP No. 14.) London, 1848. (Also in EMERSON C. KELLY, *Medical Classics,* Vol. IV, pp. 1ff. Baltimore, 1939. Kelly's *Medical Classics* differs from the other source books in giving either complete treatises or selections sufficiently long to be worth while.)

Salernum, The School of (Regimen Sanitatis Salernitanum). Trans. by JOHN HARRINGTON and ed. by R. F. PACKARD. New York, 1920.

STRABO. *Hortulus.* Trans. by R. S. LAMBERT. London, 1924.

Syriac Anatomy, Pathology and Therapeutics or *The Book of Medicine.* Trans. by E. A. WALLIS BUDGE. 2 vols. London, 1913.

THEODORIC. *Surgery.* Trans. by E. CAMPBELL and J. COLTON. 2 vols. New York, 1955–60.

CHAPTER 9

A survey of the anatomical developments in this period will be found in CHARLES SINGER, *Evolution of Anatomy* (New York, 1925; reprinted by Dover). A good summary of the syphilis discussion is carried in RIESMAN, *Medicine in the Middle Ages,* previously cited. The excellent sourcebook of R. HUNTER and J. MCALPINE: *Three Hundred years of Psychiatry, 1935–1960* (London, 1963), also begins in this period.

Illuminative biographies for this period are WALTER PAGEL, *Paracelsus* (Basel, 1958); Ch. D. O'MALLEY, *Andreas Vesalius* (Berkeley, 1964); SIR CHARLES SHERRINGTON, *The Endeavour of Jean Fernel* (Cambridge, 1946); H. M. PAECHTER, *Paracelsus* (New York, 1951); HARVEY W. CUSHING, *A Bio-bibliography of Andreas Vesalius* (New York, 1943); JEROME P. WEBSTER and M. T. GNUDI, *The Life and Times of Gaspare Tagliacozzi* (New York, 1950); and F. R. PACKARD, *Life and Times of Ambroise Paré* (New York, 1921). Packard's book contains a translation of Paré's "Apology."

Translations and Reprints

AGRICOLA. *De re metallica.* Trans. by H. C. and L. H. HOOVER. London, 1912; reprinted by Dover, 1950.

ALDROVANDI. *On Chickens.* Trans. by L. R. LIND. Norman, 1963.

Aneurism, Observations on. (Galen, Aetius, Fernelius, Paré, Guillemeau, Sennert, Hildanus, Wiseman, Lancisi, Monro, Petit, Haller, Hunter, Ballie, etc.) Trans. by J. E. ERICKSEN. (SSP No. 5.) London, 1844.

BENIVIENI, A. *On the Hidden Causes of Diseases.* Trans. by CH. SINGER. Springfield, 1954.

BERENGARIO DA CARPI, J. *A Short Introduction to Anatomy.* Trans. by L. R. LIND. Chicago, 1959.

BRIGHT, T. *A Treatise of Melancholie* (1586). Introduction by H. CRAIG. New York, 1940.

Caius, The Works of John. Ed. by E. S. ROBERTS. Cambridge, 1912. (Contains his treatise on the English Sweat. The same reprinted in Scholars Facsimiles. New York, 1937.)

CARDANO, GIROLAMO. *The Book of My Life.* Trans. by J. STONER. New York, 1930.

CLOWES, W. *Profitable and necessarie booke of observations.* Scholars Facs. New York, 1945.

CORNARO, L. *The Art of Living Long.* Milwaukee, 1905.

COYTER, VOLCHER. "Tables of the Human Body," *Op. sel. Neerl. de arte med.* XVIII, Amsterdam, 1955.

DU LAURENS, ANDRÉ. *A Discourse on the Preservation of Sight, of Melancholike Diseases* (1519). Introduction by S. V. LARKEY. (Shakespeare Assoc. Facs. No. 15.) Oxford, 1938.

ELYOT, SIR THOMAS. *The Castel of Helthe.* Scholars Facs. New York, 1937.

FRACASTORO, G. *De Contagione.* Trans. by W. C. WRIGHT. New York, 1930.

———. *Syphilis.* Trans. by VAN WYCK. Los Angeles, 1931.

Influenza in Great Britain, Annals of, 1510–1837. Ed. by THOMAS THOMPSON. (SSP No. 20.) London, 1852.

LEONARDO DA VINCI. *On the Human Body.* The anatomical, physiological and embryological drawings with translation and introduction by C. D. O'MALLEY and J. B. DE C. M. SAUNDERS. New York, 1953.

MAJOR, R. H. *Classic Descriptions of Disease.* Springfield, Ill., 1945. (Contains numerous sixteenth-century pieces by Leoniceno, Baillou, Cardano, Plater, Fernel, Lange, Botallo, etc.)

Malleus Maleficarum. Trans. by REV. M. SUMMERS. London, 1928.

MONARDES, N. *Joyfull Newes out of the Newe Founde World.* Reprint. London and New York, 1925. (On drugs found by the Spaniards in America.)

PARACELSUS. *Four Treatises.* Trans. by C. L. TEMKIN, G. ROSEN, G. ZILBOORG, and H. E. SIGERIST. Baltimore, 1941.

———. *Volumen medicinae Paramirum.* Trans. by K. F. LEIDECKER. Baltimore, 1949.

Paré, A., Selections from the Work of. Trans. by D. W. SINGER. London, 1924.

PHAIRE, TH. *The Boke of Children* (1545). Edinburgh, 1955.

SERVETUS, MICHAEL. *Non-theological Writings.* Trans. by CH. D. O'MALLEY. Philadelphia, 1953.

VESALIUS, ANDREAS. Translation of introduction to "Fabrica" in L. Clendening, *Sourcebook of Medical History.* New York, 1942.

———. *The Bloodletting letter of 1539.* Trans. by J. B. DE C. M. SAUNDERS and C. D. O'MALLEY. London, n.d.

———. *The Epitome.* Trans. by L. R. LIND. New York, 1949.

———. *On the Human Brain.* Trans. by CH. SINGER. London, 1952.

Vesalius, Illustrations from the Works of. Ed. by SAUNDERS and O'MALLEY. Cleveland, 1950.

CHAPTER 10

For an excellent appreciation of the development of physiology during the sixteenth and later centuries, read SIR MICHAEL FOSTER, *Lectures on the History of Physiology During the 16th, 17th, and 18th Centuries* (Cambridge, 1901), which also contains many original quotations. Even better is K. E. ROTSCHUH, *History of Physiology*, trans. by G. B. RISSE (Huntington, 1973). For embryology, see A. W. MEYER, *The Rise of Embryology* (Stanford, 1939). More specialized are M. ORNSTEIN, *The Role of Scientific Societies in the Seventeenth Century* (Chicago, 1928) and a paper by E. H. ACKERKNECHT, "The History of Legal Medicine," appearing in *Ciba Symposia*, Vol. II, No. 7 (Summit, N. J., 1951).

In the field of biography, WALTER PAGEL, one of the most original researchers in the field, has contributed an excellent appraisal of Van Helmont in his book, *The Religious and Philosophical Aspects of Van Helmont's Science and Medicine* (Baltimore, 1944). Other worthwhile biographies are L. T. MORE, *The Life and Works of the Honourable Robert Boyle* (New York, 1944); D. RIESMAN, *Thomas Sydenham* (New York, 1926); SIR D'ARCY POWER, *William Harvey* (London, 1898); L. CHAUVOIS, *William Harvey* (New York, 1966); and H. R. ISLER, *Thomas Willis* (New York, 1966).

Translations and Reprints

BONTEKOE, C. "Treatise about Tea." *Op. sel. Neerl. de arte med.* XIV, Amsterdam, 1937.

BONTIUS, J. "On Tropical Medicine." *Ibid.*, X, Amsterdam, 1931.

DIETZ, MASTER JOHANNES. *Autobiography*. London, 1923.

DOBELL, CLIFFORD. *Antony Van Leeuwenhoek and his "Little Animals."* New York, 1932; reprinted by Dover, 1960.

FABRICIUS OF AQUAPENDENTE. *Embryological Treatises*. Trans. by H. ADELMAN. Ithaca, N.Y., 1942.

———. *De venarum ostiolis*. Trans. by H. J. FRANKLIN. Baltimore, 1932.

HARVEY, W. *Exercitatio anatomica de motu cordis*. Trans. by CH. D. LEAKE. Springfield and Baltimore, 1931. (Also in the excellent sourcebook of F. A. WILLIUS and THOMAS E. KEYS. *Cardiac Classics*. St. Louis, 1941. Pp. 19ff.)

Harvey, The Works of. Trans. by R. WILLIS. (SSP No. 10.) London, 1847; see also Everyman's Library, No. 262. New York, 1923.

HOOKE, R. *Micrographia*. Oxford, 1938. (Vol. 13 of R. T. GUNTHER's "Early Science in Oxford"; reprinted by Dover, 1961.)

LANCISI, G. M. *Aneurisms*. Trans. by W. C. Wright. New York, 1952.

Leeuwenhoek, The Collected Letters of Antoni Van. Part I. Amsterdam, Swets & Zeitlinger, 1939.

Leeuwenhoek Letter, The (Oct. 9, 1676, to Henry Oldenberg). Trans. by BARNETT COHEN. Soc. of Amer. Bacteriologists. Baltimore, 1937.

LOWER, R. *De Catharris.* Trans. by R. HUNTER and IDA MACALPINE. London, 1963.

———. *De Corde.* Oxford, 1932. (Vol. 9 of R. T. GUNTHER's "Early Science in Oxford.")

MALPIGHI, M. *De pulmonibus observationes anatomicae.* Trans. by J. YOUNG (in *Proc. Roy. Soc. Med.*). London, 1929–1930. 23: 1ff. (Also in WILLIUS and KEYS, pp. 92ff.)

MAYOW, J. *Medico-Physical Works.* Translation of "Tractatus Quinque Medico-Phisici." Edinburgh, 1907.

PISO, W. "Medicine of the West Indies," *Op. sel. Neerl. de arte med.* XIV, Amsterdam, 1937.

RAMAZZINI, B. *De morbis artificium diatriba* (Diseases of Workers). Trans. by W. H. WRIGHT. Chicago, 1940 (also Hafner, No. 23).

STENO, N. A. *Dissertation on the Anatomy of Brain.* Copenhagen, 1950.

SYDENHAM, THOMAS. *Selections.* Trans. by J. D. COMRIE. London and New York, 1922. (Also in E. KELLY, *Medical Classics*, Vol. IV, pp. 286ff.)

TEN RHYNE, W. "Treatise on the Asiatic Leprosy." *Op. sel. Neerl. de arte med.* XIV, Amsterdam, 1937.

Selections from most of the seventeenth-century clinicians mentioned, such as Kirchner, Sylvius, Morton, Tulp, Willis, Sydenham, Sennert, Vieussens, Lower, Lancisi, and others, can be found in R. MAJOR's source book, *Classic Descriptions.* See also WILLIUS and KEYS, *Cardiac Classics.*

CHAPTER 11

FOSTER's *Lectures,* recommended for Chapter 10, is also a good source for eighteenth-century physiological developments. For pathology see ESMOND LONG, *History of Pathology* (Chicago, 1928, reprinted by Dover, 1965). J. D. COMRIE, *History of Scottish Medicine* (2 vols., London, 1929) is a good study for that country at the height of its medical fame. For a broader survey see A. WOLF, *History of Science, Technology and Philosophy in the 18th Century* (London, 1938).

Biographies of this period include W. R. AYKROYD, *Three Philosophers* (London, 1935), dealing with Lavoisier, Priestley, and Cavendish. For the Hunter brothers, see G. C. PEACHY, *A Memoir on William and John Hunter.* Also recommended are L. BAUMGARTNER, *John Howard (1726–1790)* (J. H. C., Baltimore, 1939), a bibliography with an introduction by A. M. MUIRHEAD; R. H. FOX, *Dr. John Fothergill and His Friends* (London, 1919); J. J. ABRAHAM, *Lettsom, His Life, Time, . . .* (London, 1933); L. H. RODDIS, *William Withering* (New York, 1936), and also his *James Lind* (New York, 1950). See also G. A. LINDEBOOM, *Herman Boerhaave* (London, 1968).

Translations and Reprints

Starting with the eighteenth century many medical books are no longer written in Latin, but in the vernacular. Thus you might find some such originals in your library and need not look exclusively for the reprints or translations of this list.

ANDRY, N. *Orthopedy.* Philadelphia, 1961.

ARNOLD, THOMAS. *Observations in Insanity.* Reprint. Arno Press. New York, 1976.

AUENBRUGGER, L. *On Percussion of the Chest.* Baltimore, 1936. (In the Classics Series of the Johns Hopkins Institute of the History of Medicine, abbreviated J. H. C.)

BAILLIE, M. *Morbid Anatomy.* Edited by A. E. RODIN. Springfield, 1973.

BAKER, G. *An Essay on the Endemic Colic of Devonshire.* Reprint. 1958.

BATTIE, W. *A Treatise on Madness.* Reprint. London, 1962.

CAMPER, P. "Travel Journals," *Op. sel. Neerl. de arte med.* XV, Amsterdam, 1939.

FAUCHARD, P. *The Surgeon Dentist or Treatise on the Teeth.* Trans. by L. LINDSEY. London, 1947.

FAUST, B. *Catechism of Health.* Reprint. Arno Press. New York, 1972.

FOTHERGILL, J. Selections in E. KELLY's *Classics,* Vol. V, pp. 46 ff.

HALES, STEPHEN. Selections in WILLIUS and KEYS, *Classics,* pp. 131 ff.

———. *Statistical Essays.* Hafner No. 22.

HALLER, A. VON. *A Dissertation on the Sensible and Irritable Parts of Animals.* Trans. by O. TEMKIN. Baltimore, 1936. (J.H.C.)

HASLAM, J. *Observations on Madness.* Reprint. Arno Press. New York, 1976.

HEBERDEN, W. *An Introduction to the Study of Physics.* Reprint by LE ROY CRUMMER. New York, 1929.

———. *Commentaries.* Hafner No. 18.

Hewson, W., Works of. (SSP No. 8.) Reprint. London, 1844.

HUNTER, J. Selections in E. KELLY's *Classics,* Vol. IV, pp. 400 ff.

JENNER, E. *An Inquiry into the Causes and Effects of the Variolae Vaccinae.* Reprint. Milan, 1923.

LIND, J. *Treatise on Scurvy.* Reprint. Edinburgh, 1953.

———. *The Health of Seamen.* Greenwich, 1965.

MORGAGNI, G. B. Selections in KELLY's *Classics,* Vol. IV, pp. 628 ff.

———. *The Seats and Causes of Diseases.* Hafner No. 13.

Observations on Surgical Diseases of the Head and Neck. Selected from the Memoirs of the Royal Academy of Surgery of France. Trans. by D. OTTLEY. (SSP No. 13.) London, 1848.

PARKINSON, J. *An Essay on the Shaking Palsy.* Reprint. London, 1959.

PARRY, C. H. Selections in KELLY's *Classics,* Vol. V.

PERCIVAL, THOMAS. *Medical Ethics.* Reprint, with introduction by CHAUNCEY D. LEAKE. Baltimore, 1927.

PERFECT, W. *Annals of Insanity.* Reprint. Arno Press. New York, 1976.
PINEL, P. *A Treatise on Insanity.* Hafner No. 14.
POTT, P. Selections in E. KELLY's *Classics,* Vol. I, pp. 271 ff.
SMELLIE, W. *Treatise on Midwifery.* 2 vols. (NSSP No. 68.) London, 1876.
WITHERING, W. Selections in E. KELLY's *Classics,* Vol. II, pp. 294 ff.
  For other clinicians (Huxham, Tronchin, Perry, Cotugno, etc.) see again MAJOR's *Classic Descriptions.*

CHAPTER 12

One of the best medicohistorical books ever written is KNUD FABER, *Nosography* (New York, 1930), a history of clinical medicine, mainly nineteenth century. An interesting social history of medicine in this same period is R. H. SHRYOCK, *The Development of Modern Medicine* (New York, 1947). See also ERWIN H. ACKERKNECHT, *Medicine in the Paris Hospital 1794–1848* (Baltimore, 1966), and ERNA LESKY, *The Vienna Medical School in the 19th Century* (Baltimore, 1976).

Translations and Reprints

ADAMS, R. Selections in KELLY's *Classics,* Vol. III, pp. 620 ff.
ADDISON, THOMAS. Selections in *ibid.,* Vol. II, pp. 233 ff.
———. *Collected Works.* (NSSP No. 36.) London, 1868.
BELL, CHARLES. Selections in KELLY's *Classics,* Vol. I, pp. 81 ff.
BRETONNEAU, GUERSANT, TROUSSEAU. *Memoirs on Diphtheria.* Trans. by R. H. SEMPLE. (NSSP No. 3.) London, 1859.
BRIGHT, R. *Abdominal Tumors.* (NSSP No. 6.) London, 1860.
BRODIE, B. C. Selections in KELLY's *Classics,* Vol. II, pp. 882 ff.
BURNS, A. *Observations on Diseases of the Heart.* Hafner No. 21.
CHEYNE, J. Selections in *ibid.,* Vol. III, pp. 698 ff.
COLLES, A. Selections in *ibid.,* Vol. IV, pp. 1026 ff.
———. *Selected Works.* (NSSP No. 92.) London, 1881.
CORRIGAN, D. J. Selections in KELLY's *Classics,* Vol. I, pp. 673 ff.; also in WILLIUS and KEYS' source book.
CORVISART, N. *An Essay on the Diseases of the Heart.* Hafner No. 16.
DUPUYTREN, G. Selections in *ibid.,* Vol. IV, pp. 86 ff.
———. *Lesions of the Vascular System and Other Surgical Complications.* Trans. by F. LE GROS CLARK. (SSP No. 23.) London, 1854.
———. *On the Diseases of Bones.* Trans. by F. LE GROS CLARK. (SSP No. 9.) London, 1857.
GRAVES, R. *Lectures on the Practice of Clinical Medicine.* 2 vols. (NSSP No. 109.) London, 1884.
———. Selections in KELLY's *Classics,* Vol. V, pp. 22 ff.
HODGKIN, THOMAS. Selections in *ibid.,* Vol. I, pp. 731 ff.
LAENNEC. *Selections.* Trans. by SIR W. H. WHITE. London, 1923.
———. *A Treatise on the Diseases of the Chest.* Hafner No. 17.

Louis, P. C. A. *Researches on Phthisis.* Trans. by W. H. WALSHE. (SSP No. 2.) London, 1844.
STOKES, W. *Diseases of the Chest.* (NSSP No. 98.) London, 1882.
——. Selections in KELLY's *Classics,* Vol. III, pp. 710 ff.
TROUSSEAU, A. *Lectures on Clinical Medicine.* Trans. by P. V. BAZIRE. 3 vols. (NSSP No. 35.) London, 1882.
VELPEAU, A. *Diseases of the Breast.* Trans. by M. HENRY. London, 1854.

For nineteenth-century clinicians see also MAJOR's *Classic Descriptions.*

CHAPTER 13

A good general survey is R. H. SHRYOCK, *The Development of Modern Medicine* (New York, 1947). For the story of pathology, see ESMOND R. LONG, *A History of Pathology* (Baltimore, 1928, reprinted by Dover, 1965). The "Clio Medica Series" offers a number of short, authoritative histories pertinent to this period, including G. W. CORNER, *Anatomy* (New York, 1931); J. F. Fulton, *Physiology* (New York, 1931); GRAHAM LUSK, *Nutrition* (New York, 1933); and E. B. KRUMBHAAR, *Pathology* (New York, 1937). Hafner has fortunately reprinted *Clio medica* in recent years. MEYER's *Rise of Embryology,* cited for Chapter 10, is also good for the developments in histology and embryology in this period. A special study of note is T. BILLROTH, *The Medical Sciences in the German Universities* (New York, 1924).

J. M. D. OLMSTED has contributed three notable biographies of men in this period: *Claude Bernard* (New York, 1928); *François Magendie* (New York, 1945); and *Charles-Édouard Brown-Séquard* (Baltimore, 1946). T. H. BAST has written a number of worth-while biographical essays on German nineteenth-century anatomists—Koelliker, Schultze, etc.—published mainly in the *Annals of Medical History* (see Index of *Annals*). For a life of Henle see VICTOR ROBINSON, *Life of Jacob Henle* (New York, 1921). For Virchow see E. H. ACKERKNECHT, *Rudolf Virchow* (Madison, Wis., 1953). For Valentin, Gruby, Remak, and Auerbach see BRUNO KISCH, *Forgotten Leaders of Modern Medicine* (Philadelphia, 1954). For Broca see F. SCHILLER, *Paul Broca* (Berkeley, 1979). Also recommended are the sourcebook by B. H. WILLIER and J. OPPENHEIMER, *Foundations of Experimental Embryology* (Englewood Cliffs, 1964), and the essay collection, *The Historical Development of Physiological Thought,* edited by PAUL F. CRANEFIELD and C. McC. BROOKS (New York, 1959). Also important are PAUL F. CRANEFIELD, *The Way in and the Way out: François Magendie, Charles Bell, and the Roots of the Spinal Nerves,* Futura Publishing Company (Mount Kisco, 1975); O. TEMKIN, *The Double Face of Janus and Other Essays in the History of Medicine* (Baltimore, 1977); and M. A. FLORKIN, *History of Biochemistry,* 4 vols. (Amsterdam, 1972–1974).

Translations and Reprints

BELL, CHARLES. Selections in KELLY's *Classics*, Vol. I, pp. 81 ff.

BERNARD, C. *An Introduction to the Study of Experimental Medicine*. Trans. by H. C. GREENE. New York, 1927 (also reprinted by Dover).

——. Selections in KELLY's *Classics*, Vol. III, pp. 512 ff.

BERT, P. *Barometric Pressure*. Trans. by M. A. and F. A. HITCHCOCK. Columbus, 1943.

BERTHOLD, A. A. "The Transplantation of Testes," *Bull. Hist. Med.* 16: 399–401, 1944.

BINZ, K. *Lectures on Pharmacology*. Trans. by A. C. LATHAM. (NSSP No. 154.) London, 1895.

COHNHEIM, J. *Lectures on General Pathology*. Trans. by A. B. MC-KEE. 3 vols. (NSSP No. 126.) London, 1887.

HELMHOLTZ, H. *Mechanism of the Ossicles of the Ear.* (NSSP No. 62.) London, 1874.

——. *On Thought in Medicine*. Baltimore, 1938. (J. H. C.)

——. *On the Sense of Tone*. Reprint. (Dover.)

——. *A Treatise on Physiological Optics*. Reprint. (Dover.)

HENLE, J. *On Miasmata and Contagia*. Trans. by GEORGE ROSEN. Baltimore, 1938. (J. H. C.)

KOELLIKER, A. *A Manual of Human Histology*. Trans. by G. BUSH and THOMAS HUXLEY. 2 vols. (SSP No. 22.) London, 1853.

ROKITANSKY, C. *Pathological Anatomy*. Trans. by W. A. SWAINE. 4 vols. (SSP No. 17.) London, 1849.

SCHWANN, THOMAS. *Microscopic Researches*. Trans. by H. SMITH. (SSP No. 12.) London, 1847.

VIRCHOW, R. *Cellular Pathology*. Trans. by F. CHANCE. Philadelphia, 1860.

CHAPTER 14

FABER's *Nosography,* cited for Chapter 12, is also excellent for this period.

Translations and Reprints

EWALD, C. A. *Lectures on Diseases of the Digestive Organs*. Trans. by R. SAUNBY. 2 vols. (NSSP No. 136.) London, 1891.

FRERICHS, F. THOMAS. *A Clinical Treatise on Diseases of the Liver*. Trans. by MURCHISON. 2 vols. (NSSP No. 7.) London, 1860.

KUSSMAUL, A., and A. TENNER. *On Epileptiform Convulsions Caused by Profuse Bleedings*. Trans. by E. BRONNER. (NSSP No. 5.) London, 1859.

NAUNYN, B. *A Treatise on Cholelithiasis*. Trans. by A. E. GARROD. (NSSP No. 158.) London, 1896.

OSLER, SIR WILLIAM. Selections in KELLY's *Classics*, Vol. IV, pp. 174 ff.

WUNDERLICH, C. A. *On Temperature in Diseases*. Trans. by W. B. WOODMAN. (NSSP No. 49.) London, 1871.

See also MAJOR's *Classic Descriptions* for passages from Kussmaul, Minkowski, Quincke, McKenzie, Osler, etc.

CHAPTER 15

For the best account of the rise of the science of bacteriology, see W. BULLOCH, *The History of Bacteriology* (London, 1938). There are several biographies of Pasteur available. Also recommended is the sourcebook on virology by N. HAHON (Englewood Cliffs, 1964), and R. HOEPPLI, *Parasites and Parasitic Diseases in Early Medicine* (Singapore, 1959).

Translations and Reprints

COHN, F. *Bacteria*. Trans. by M. LEIKIND. Baltimore, 1939. (J. H. C.)

FINLAY, J. C. Selections in KELLY's *Classics*, Vol. II, pp. 540 ff.

KOCH, R. Selections in *ibid.*, Vol. II, p. 714.

——. *Investigations into the Etiology of Traumatic Infective Diseases*. Trans. by W. W. CHEYNE. (NSSP No. 88.) London, 1880.

——, LOEFFLER, GAFFKY, EBERTH, NEISSER *et al*. Bacteria in Relation to Disease. (NSSP No. 115.) London, 1886. (Collection of important monographs.)

KUECHENMEISTER, F. *On Animal and Vegetable Parasites of the Human Body*. Trans. by E. LANKESTER. 2 vols. (SSP No. 28.) London, 1857.

LAVERAN, A. *Paludism*. Trans. by J. W. MARTIN. (NSSP No. 146.) London, 1893.

MARCHIAFAVA, E., A. BIGNAMI, and J. MANNABERG. *Two Monographs on Malaria*. (NSSP No. 150.) London, 1894.

SMITH, THEOBALD. Selections in KELLY's *Classics*, Vol. I, pp. 314 ff.

WELCH, W. H. Selections in *ibid.*, Vol. V, pp. 822 ff.

CHAPTER 16

For a general survey of medicine in modern times see C. D. HAAGENSEN and W. E. B. LLOYD, *A Hundred Years of Medicine* (New York, 1943), which is particularly good on surgery. See also the book by the WANGENSTEENS and R. G. RICHARDSON, *History of Modern Surgery* (1964). SIR D'ARCY POWER has written *A Short History of Surgery* (London, 1933). E. JAMESON, *Gynecology and Obstetrics* (New York, 1936) is another of the concise, authoritative histories in the "Clio Medica" series. See also J. V. RICCI, *The Development of Gynaecological Surgery and Instruments* (Philadelphia, 1949). For the history of anesthesia, use the "History" by THOMAS E. KEYS (New York, 1945; reprinted by Dover) and the sourcebook, *Foundations of Anesthesiology*, by A. FAULCONER, JR., and THOMAS E. KEYS (2 vols., Springfield, 1965).

There are a number of recent popular biographies available for this period, including SEALE HARRIS' excellent *Woman's Surgeon, the Life of J. M. Sims* (New York, 1950); F. SLAUGHTER, *Immortal Magyar: Semmelweis* (New York, 1950); K. B. ABSOLOM, *Theodor Billroth* (Lawrence, 1979); and D. GUTHRIE, *Lord Lister* (Baltimore, 1949).

Translations and Reprints

BILLROTH, THEODOR. *Lectures on Surgical Pathology and Therapy.* 2 vols. (NSSP No. 73.) London, 1877.

———. *Clinical Surgery.* Trans. by C. T. DENT. (NSSP No. 94.) London, 1889.

FITZ, R. H. Selections in KELLY's *Classics,* Vol. II, pp. 446 ff.

HALSTED, W. S. Selections in *ibid.,* Vol. III, pp. 384 ff.

HOLMES, O. W. Selections in *ibid.,* Vol. I, pp. 195 ff.

LISTER, LORD JOSEPH. Selections in *ibid.,* Vol. II, pp. 4 ff.

———. *Six Papers.* Selected by SIR RICKMAN J. GODLEY. London, 1912.

MCBURNEY, CHARLES. Selections in KELLY's *Classics,* Vol. II, pp. 492 ff.

MCDOWELL, E. Selections in *ibid.,* Vol. II, pp. 642 ff.

MIKULICZ-RADECKI, J. VON. Selections in *ibid.,* Vol. II, pp. 106 ff.

PAGET, SIR JAMES. Selections in *ibid.,* Vol. I, pp. 5 ff.

POZZI, S. *A Treatise on Gynecology.* 2 vols. (NSSP No. 140.) London, 1892.

SEMMELWEIS, I. P. "The Etiology of Childbed Fever" in KELLY's *Classics,* Vol. V, pp. 338 ff. (Translation of entire book.)

SIMS, J. M. Selections in *ibid.,* Vol. II, pp. 662 ff.

CHAPTER 17

For an excellent study of the development of specialization in medicine, particularly as illustrated in the field of ophthalmology, see GEORGE ROSEN, *The Specialization of Medicine* (New York, 1944), Arno Press reprint (New York, 1972). Competent surveys of pediatrics and neurology are found in two chapters by F. H. GARRISON, his "History of Pediatrics" in I. A. ABT, *A System of Pediatrics* (Philadelphia, 1923), Vol. I., pp. 1–170; and his "History of Neurology" in C. L. DANA, *Textbook of Nervous Disorders* (10th ed.; New York, 1925), pp. iv–liii: also published separately and edited by MCHENRY (1969). Valuable reference books are W. HAYMAKER and F. SCHILLER, *The Founders of Neurology* (Springfield, 1970), and O. TEMKIN's classic *The Falling Sickness* (Baltimore, 1971). The best history of modern psychotherapy is H. F. ELLENBERGER, *The Discovery of the Unconscious* (New York, 1970). Recommended sourcebooks are TINTEROW, *Classics in Hypnosis* (Springfield, 1970); IMMERGUT, *Classic Articles in Urology* (Springfield, 1967); and G.

BALLESTER, et al., *Classics in Otology* (London, 1978). Also recommended are F. A. WILLIUS and T. J. DRY, *A History of the Heart and Circulation* (Philadelphia, 1948). For a historical understanding of orthopedics, see E. M. BICK, *Sourcebook of Orthopedics* (Baltimore, 1937). Two short texts available on the history of psychiatry are E. H. ACKERKNECHT, *A Short History of Psychiatry* (London and New York, 1959), and J. M. SCHNECK, *A History of Psychiatry* (Springfield, 1960). An excellent sourcebook for British developments is R. HUNTER and IDA MACALPINE, *Three Hundred Years of Psychiatry 1535–1860* (London, 1963). For treatment of other specialties, see B. CHANCE, *Ophthalmology* (New York, 1939); JONATHAN WRIGHT, *History of Laryngology and Rhinology* (2d ed.; Philadelphia, 1914), and HAAGENSEN and LLOYD, *A Hundred Years of Medicine,* mentioned already for its treatment of surgery.

Translations and Reprints

BLEULER, EUGEN. *Psychiatry.* Reprint. Arno Press. New York, 1976.

CHARCOT, J. M. *Diseases of the Nervous System.* Trans. by G. SIGERSON. 2 vols. (NSSP No. 72.) London, 1875 (also Hafner No. 19).

———. *Localisation of Cerebral and Spinal Disease.* Trans. by W. B. HADDEN. (NSSP No. 102.) London, 1883.

———. *Lectures on Senile Diseases.* Trans. by W. S. TUKE. (NSSP No. 95.) London, 1881. (Interesting introductory lecture on medicine in general.)

CZERMAK, J. N. *On the Laryngoscope.* Trans. by D. GIBB. (NSSP No. 11.) London, 1866.

DONDERS, F. C. *On the Anomalies of Accommodation and Refraction of the Eye.* Trans. by W. D. MOORE. (NSSP No. 22.) London, 1864.

DUCHENNE, G. *Selected Works.* Trans. by C. V. POORE. (NSSP No. 105.) London, 1883.

ESQUIROL, J. E. D. *Mental Maladies.* Hafner No. 25.

FEUCHTERSLEBEN, E. VON. *Principles of Medical Psychology.* Trans. by H. E. LLOYD. (SSP No. 11.) London, 1847.

GRAEFE, A. VON. *Iridectomy.* Trans. by TH. WINDSOR. (NSSP No. 5.) London, 1859.

GRIESINGER, W. *Mental Pathology and Therapeutics.* Trans. by C. C. ROBERTSON. (NSSP No. 33.) London, 1882 (also Hafner No. 26).

HEBRA, F. *Diseases of the Skin.* Trans. by C. H. FAGGE. 5 vols. (NSSP No. 30.) London, 1860.

HENOCH, E. *Children's Diseases.* Trans. by J. THOMPSON. 2 vols. (NSSP No. 125.) London, 1889.

HUTCHINSON, SIR JONATHAN. *Diseases of the Skin.* (NSSP No. 40.) London, 1869.

———. Selections in KELLY's *Classics,* Vol. V, pp. 108 ff.

JACKSON, J. HUGHLINGS. Selections in *ibid.,* Vol. III, pp. 898 ff.

———. *Selected Writings.* 2 vols. London, 1937.

JANET, P. *Psychological Healing.* Reprint. Arno Press. New York, 1976.

KRAEPELIN, E. *Manic-depressions. Paranoia.* Reprint. Arno Press. New York, 1976.

MARIE, PIERRE. *Acromegaly.* (NSSP No. 137.) London, 1891.

———. *Diseases of the Spinal Cord.* Trans. by M. LUBBOCK. (NSSP No. 152.) London, 1895.

ROMBERG, M. *Nervous Diseases of Man.* Trans. by E. H. SIEVEKING. 2 vols. (SSP No. 21.) London, 1853.

UNNA, G. *Selected Writings.* Trans. by P. S. ABRAHAM. (NSSP No. 143.) London, 1893.

CHAPTER 18

In addition to SHRYOCK, *Development of Modern Medicine,* and HAAGENSEN and LLOYD, *A Hundred Years of Medicine,* see C.-E. A. WINSLOW, *The Conquest of Epidemic Disease* (Princeton, 1943), an excellent survey of the progress made in that field during the nineteenth century. The best single history of public health is that by GEORGE ROSEN (New York, 1958). Much material can be found in R. SAND, *The Advance to Social Medicine* (London, 1952).

Two interesting biographies pertinent to this period are E. E. HUME, *Max von Pettenkofer* (New York, 1927), and M. GORGAS, *W. C. Gorgas* (Garden City, N. Y., 1924). In addition M. WALKER, *Pioneers of Public Health* (London, 1930) contains biographic sketches of most of the leaders of the public health movement. For the history of women in medicine see KATE C. HURD MEAD, *A History of Women in Medicine* (Haddam, 1938).

Translations and Reprints

BUDD, W. *Typhoid Fever.* Reprint. New York, 1931.

CHADWICK, EDWIN. *The Health of Nations.* London.

PANUM, P. L. *Observations Made During an Epidemic of Measles.* Reprint. New York, 1940. Also in KELLY's *Classics,* Vol. III, pp. 803 ff.

PETTENKOFER, M. VON. *The Value of Health to a City.* Trans. by H. E. SIGERIST. Baltimore, 1941. (J. H. C.)

SHATTUCK, LEMUEL. *Report.* Reprinted in J. C. WHIPPLE. *State Sanitation.* Cambridge, Mass., 1917.

SNOW, J. *On Cholera.* Reprint. New York, 1936.

THACKRAH, CH. T. *The effects of arts, trades and professions on health and longevity.* Reprinted in A. MEIKLEJOHN, *Ch. T. Thackrah.* Edinburgh, 1957.

CHAPTER 19

The classic reference for United States medical history is F. R. PACKARD, *History of Medicine in the U. S.* (2 vols., 2d ed.; New York,

1931). For a short competent survey, see H. E. SIGERIST, *American Medicine* (New York, 1934). For a more recent survey, see H. BORDLEY and A. HARVEY, *Two Centuries of American Medicine* (Philadelphia, 1976). A special aspect of American medicine is covered in R. H. SHRYOCK, *American Medical Research, Past and Present* (New York, 1947). For medical education, read ABRAHAM FLEXNER's classic report, *Medical Education in the U. S. and Canada* (New York, 1910). This report was influential in the renaissance of American medical education. For the earlier period see the solid work by W. F. NORWOOD, *Medical Education in the U. S. Before the Civil War* (Philadelphia, 1944). Important analyses of United States epidemics are J. H. POWELL's account of the yellow fever plague in Philadelphia in 1793, *Bring Out Your Dead* (Philadelphia, 1949), and CHARLES E. ROSENBERG, *The Cholera Years* (Chicago, 1962).

There are a multitude of biographies and autobiographies of American medical figures, some very good and many very poor. Autobiographies of medical leaders, early ones such as Rush, Caldwell, J. M. Sims, Gross, and Drake down to more recent figures such as Cannon, Alice Hamilton, and Zinsser, are worthy of exploration. Of the many biographies, at least passing reference must be paid those of Rush (by GOODMAN), Shippen (by CORNER), McDowell (by SCHACHNER), Drake (by JUETTNER), Beaumont (by MYER), Welch (by J. and S. FLEXNER), Billings (by GARRISON), Osler (by CUSHING) and Biggs (by WINSLOW). In addition W. S. MIDDLETON has published numerous biographical essays of early Philadelphia doctors in the old *Annals of Medical History*.

Reprints

BEARD, G. M. *American Nervousness.* Introduction by CHARLES ROSENBERG. Reprint. Arno Press. New York, 1972.

BEAUMONT, W. *Experiments and Observations on the Gastric Juice.* Cambridge, Mass., 1929 (reprinted by Dover, 1959).

BILLINGS, J. S. *Selected Essays.* 1965.

BLACKWELL, E. *Essays in Medical Sociology.* New York, 1972.

DRAKE, D. *Selected Writings.* Lexington, 1970.

DRAKE, DANIEL. *Essays on Medical Education in the U. S.* Introduction by D. A. TUCKER, JR. Baltimore, 1953. (J. H. C.)

FLINT, AUSTIN. Selections in KELLY's *Classics,* Vol. IV, pp. 842 ff.

McCREADY, H. W. *On the Influence of Trades in the U. S. on the Production of Disease* (1837). Introduction by GENEVIEVE MILLER. Baltimore, 1943. (J. H. C.)

MORGAN, JOHN. *Discourse upon the Institution of Medical Schools in America.* Introduction by A. FLEXNER. Baltimore, 1937. (J. H. C.)

OSLER, W. *A Way of Life* (reprinted by Dover, 1958).

RUSH, BENJAMIN. *Selected Writings.* Ed. by D. D. RUNES. New York, 1947.

———. *Medical Inquiries upon the Diseases of the Mind.* Hafner No. 15.

SMITH, NATHAN. Selections in KELLY's *Classics,* Vol. I, pp. 773 ff.

THATCHER, THOMAS. *A brief rule to guide the common people how to order themselves in the Small Pocks.* Introduction by H. R. VIETS. Baltimore, 1937. (J. H. C.)

WELCH, W. H. *Adaptation in Pathological Processes.* Introduction by S. FLEXNER. Baltimore, 1937. (J. H. C.)

WOODWARD, J. *Camp Diseases in the U.S. Army.* New York, 1964.

CHAPTER 20

See again the previously cited histories by SHRYOCK and by HAAGENSEN and LLOYD for a broad survey of twentieth-century medical developments. Three books on the history of surgery deserve special mention: L. A. HOCHBERG, *Thoracic Surgery before the 20th Century* (New York, 1960); A. HURWITZ and G. A. DEGENSHEIM, *Milestones in Modern Surgery* (New York, 1958); and A. E. WALKER, *A History of Neurological Surgery* (Baltimore, 1957). B. HOLNSTEDT and G. LILJESTRAND have published *Readings in Pharmacology* (Oxford, 1963).

There is a wealth of biographical material for the modern period. Particularly outstanding are ÈVE CURIE, *Marie Curie* (New York, 1937); O. GLASER, *Dr. W. C. Roentgen* (Springfield, Ill., 1945); J. F. FULTON, *Harvey Cushing* (Springfield, Ill., 1946); LLOYD STEVENSON, *Frederick Banting* (Toronto, 1946); JOHN ECCLES and W. C. GIBSON, *Sherrington* (New York, 1979); and *Nobel Lectures, 1901–1980* (Amsterdam). Histories of a few more recent disciplines are: A. R. BLEICH, *Story of X-Rays* (Dover, 1962), H. J. PARISH, *History of Immunization* (Edinburgh, 1965); A. H. STUERTEVANT, *History of Genetics* (New York, 1965).

Reprints

DUNBAR, F. *Emotion and Bodily Changes.* Reprint. Arno Press. New York, 1976.

GARROD, A. E. *Inborn Errors of Metabolism.* Reprint. London, 1963.

SHERRINGTON, C. S. *Selected Writings.* Oxford, 1979.

TAYLOR, J. H. *Selections of Molecular Genetics.* New York, 1969.

INDEX